Incretin Biology
A Practical Guide

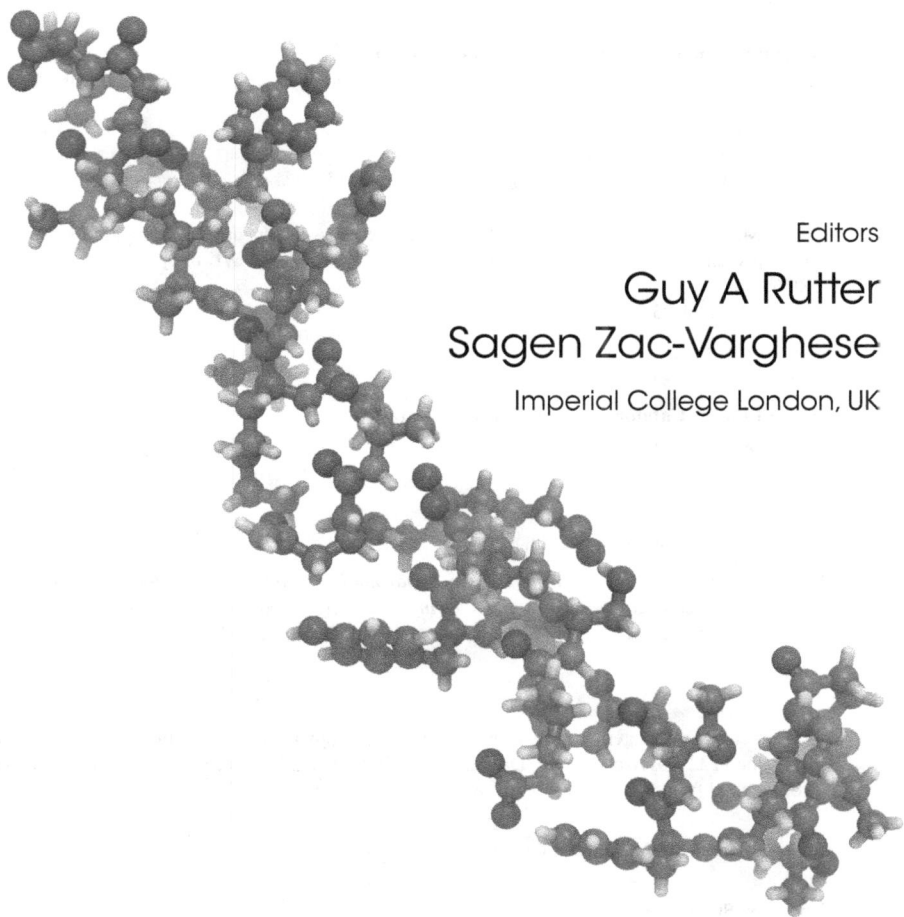

Editors

Guy A Rutter
Sagen Zac-Varghese

Imperial College London, UK

Imperial College Press

ICP

Published by

Imperial College Press
57 Shelton Street
Covent Garden
London WC2H 9HE

Distributed by

World Scientific Publishing Co. Pte. Ltd.
5 Toh Tuck Link, Singapore 596224
USA office: 27 Warren Street, Suite 401-402, Hackensack, NJ 07601
UK office: 57 Shelton Street, Covent Garden, London WC2H 9HE

Library of Congress Cataloging-in-Publication Data
Incretin biology : a practical guide : GLP-1 and GIP physiology / [edited by] Guy A. Rutter &
Sagen Zac-Varghese.
    p. ; cm.
  Includes bibliographical references.
  ISBN 978-1-78326-736-1 (alk. paper)
  I. Rutter, Guy A., editor. II. Zac-Varghese, Sagen, editor.
  [DNLM: 1. Diabetes Mellitus--drug therapy. 2. Incretins--therapeutic use. 3. Bariatric Surgery.
4. Hypoglycemic Agents--therapeutic use. 5. Incretins--physiology. WK 825]
  RC661.I6
  616.4'62061--dc23
                                        2015021097

British Library Cataloguing-in-Publication Data
A catalogue record for this book is available from the British Library.

In-house Editors: Mary Simpson/Dipasri Sardar

Typeset by Stallion Press
Email: enquires@stallionpress.com

List of Contributors

A.E. Adriaenssens (University of Cambridge)
A. Ahmed (Imperial College London)
A. Bertling (Imperial College London)
S. R. Bloom (Imperial College London)
S. C. Cork (University College London)
G. da Silva Xavier (Imperial College London)
M. Godazgar (University of Oxford)
R. Gomes-Faria (Imperial College London)
F. Gribble (University of Cambridge)
D. J. Hodson (Imperial College London)
J.J. Holst (Panum Institute, University of Copenhagen)
M. K. Holt (University College London)
L. McCulloch (University of Oxford)
A. Mondragon (Imperial College London)
R. Ramracheya (University of Oxford)
F. Reimann (University of Cambridge)
P. Rorsman (University of Oxford)
G. A. Rutter (Imperial College London)

J. E. Richards (University College London)
S. Trapp (University College London)
C. Tsironis (Imperial College London)
S. Zac-Varghese (Imperial College London)

Contents

Preface

Working together as a clinician and as a basic researcher we have felt the need for a text that may be used both as a simple reference and as a practical guide for students embarking on incretin research.

This book covers the discovery of the incretin effect; the entero-endocrine cells that produce incretin hormones; the effects of incretins on the pancreas (α and β cells) and within the central nervous system; the practical, clinical application of incretin biology for patients with type 2 diabetes and obesity; and finally, the role of incretins in bariatric surgery. It also includes unanswered questions and unmet challenges within this field.

The key contributors to this book are leaders within this field and have spent a lifetime contributing to the wealth of knowledge that now exists surrounding incretin biology. As the student will know, setting up a new protocol within a laboratory is time-consuming and can cause dilemma and consternation. Thus students may benefit from the detailed protocols, methods and helpful hints also provided here. We hope that this text will prove an invaluable resource for students and further research within this field.

G.A. Rutter
S. Zac-Varghese

Abbreviations

5-HT	5-hydroxytryptamine
α-MG	α-methylglucopyranoside
ADCY	adenylate cyclase
ADP	adenosine diphosphate
AGRP	agouti-related peptide
ARC	arcuate nucleus
ATP	adenosine triphosphate
ATP/ADP	ratio of free ATP:free ADP in the cytosol
BAC	bacterial artificial chromosome
BAT	brown adipose tissue
BBB	blood brain barrier
BMI	body mass index
BPD	biliopancreatic diversion
$[Ca^{2+}]_i$	intracellular calcium concentration;
cAMP	3′-5′-cyclic adenosine monophosphate
CCK	cholecystokinin
CFP	cerulean fluorescent protein

CICR	Ca^{2+}-induced Ca^{2+} release
DMNX	dorsal motor nucleus of the vagus
DVC	dorsal vagal complex
DS	duodenal switch
Epac	exchange of protein activated by cAMP
ERK	extracellular regulated kinase
Ex4	exendin-4
Ex9	exendin-9
FACS	fluorescent assisted cell sorting
FFA	free fatty acid
FRET	Förster resonance energy transfer
GE	genetically-encoded
GECI	genetically encoded calcium indicators
GFP	green fluorescent protein
GIP	glucose-dependent insulinotropic polypeptide
GJ	gap junction
GLP-1	glucagon-like peptide-1
GLP-1R	GLP-1 receptor
GPCR	G-protein-coupled receptor
GSIS	glucose stimulated insulin secretion
HbA1c	glycated haemoglobin
i.c.v.	intracerebroventricular
IP3	inositol (1,4,5)-triphosphate
i.v.	intravenous
JIB	jejenoileal bypass
K_{ATP}	ATP-sensitive K^+ channel
LAGB	laparoscopic adjustable gastric banding
MAPK	mitogen-activated protein kinase
NAc	nucleus accumbens
NPY	neuropeptide Y

OEA	oleoylethanolamide
OXM	oxyntomodulin
PPG	preproglucagon
PKA	protein kinase A
PKB	protein kinase B
PKC	protein kinase C
POMC	proopiomelanocortin
PVN	paraventricular nucleus
PYY	peptide tyrosine tyrosine
RFP	red fluorescent protein
RYGB	Roux en Y gastric bypass
SCFA	short chain fatty acids
SG	sleeve gastrectomy
SGLT	sodium glucose co-transporter
T2D	type 2 diabetes
TMRE	tetramethylrhodamine ethyl ester perchlorate
VDCC	voltage-dependent calcium channel
VSG	vertical sleeve gastrectomy
VTA	ventral tegmental area
YFP	yellow fluorescent protein

Useful Terms

Gene expression — the process of using a DNA template to synthesise nascent mRNA from which a gene is translated into a sequence of amino acids by ribosomal complex to make proteins.

Transgene — a foreign gene introduced into the cell.

Transduction — process of delivering a foreign gene into the target cell by a virus, typically using a viral vector.

Expression cassette — a DNA sequence encoding elements required for efficient gene expression (promoter, transgene and poly-adenylation signal).

Knock-in — insertion of an open reading frame into a genome usually of a mouse to produce a transgenic strain. For reporter genes like fluorescent proteins the ROSA26 locus is often used as a target because of few side effects and stable expression.

Lox-stop — two homotypic lox p sequences flanking a transcriptional stop sequence preventing transcription and therefore translation of the downstream encoded gene. Removal of the lox stop permits gene expression and is permanent.

Cre-recombinase — enzyme which promotes DNA recombination by recognising specific DNA sequences called lox p sites.

Bregma — the anatomical point of the skull at which the coronal suture is intersected perpendicularly by the sagittal suture.

Lambda — the point of meeting of the sagittal and lambdoid suture.

DREADDs — designer receptors exclusively activated by designer drugs. These are G-protein-coupled receptors that are only activated by CNO (clozapine-n-oxide), not found in mammals. CNO can be administered in feeding water or injected.

Chapter 1

History of Incretin Discovery and Clinical Application

S.E.K. Zac-Varghese and S.R. Bloom

Department of Investigative Medicine, Imperial College London

1.1. Introduction

In 1902, Bayliss and Starling identified and characterised the first hormone, a substance secreted into the blood stream, influencing a distant organ.[1] Prior to this, communication between organs was thought to be mediated by the nervous system. The hormone they discovered, secretin, was released by the duodenum and stimulated the exocrine pancreas, i.e. the flow of pancreatic digestive enzymes. Starling postulated that a similar duodenal substance might also stimulate pancreatic endocrine function. Almost thirty years later, La Barre and Still discovered that crude secretin contained two fractions, one that stimulated the exocrine pancreas and the other the endocrine pancreas; this fraction lowered blood glucose.[2] La Barre coined the term "incretin" for a substance produced from upper gastrointestinal tract that lowered blood glucose. The *incretin effect* is defined as the greater insulin release after an oral compared to an intravenous glucose load (Fig. 1.1). Half of the insulin secreted after an oral glucose load is stimulated by gastrointestinal factors, and in 1969

1

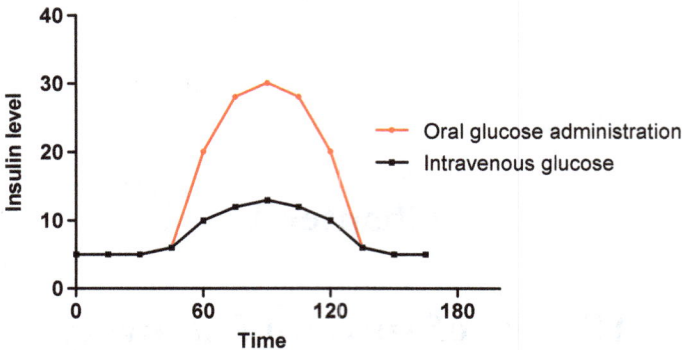

Figure 1.1. Graph of the incretin effect. Insulin levels in response to oral and intravenous glucose loads. The difference between the two responses is known as the incretin effect, the increased secretion of insulin with an oral compared to intravenous glucose load.

Unger and Eisentraut coined the term "entero-insular axis".[3] This term encompasses all the signals arising from the gut that influence the release of hormones from the pancreas.

1.2. Discovery of GIP

In 1970, John C. Brown sequenced a new peptide hormone, gastric inhibitory peptide (GIP), a 42-amino-acid peptide released mainly from entero-endocrine K cells in the duodenum, and also the hippocampus.[4] The tissue specific prohormone convertase, PC2, converts GIP_{1-42} into active GIP_{1-30}. The human GIP gene is located on the long arm of chromosome 17. GIP was initially found to have an inhibitory effect on gastric acid secretion. Later, the insulinotropic effect of GIP was determined and the acronym was changed to "glucose-dependent insulinotropic peptide". Studies using antibodies against GIP (blocking the action of GIP) demonstrated that additional hormones contributed to the incretin effect. In addition, in patients with small bowel resection, the incretin effect was still present. This led to the hypothesis that an alternate incretin hormone existed that originated from the large intestine.

1.3. Discovery of GLP-1

In 1983, glucagon like peptide-1 (GLP-1) was identified by cloning preproglucagon.[5] Preproglucagon is a 180-amino-acid peptide expressed by: Pancreatic α cells, entero-endocrine L and some K cells, and in the brain, in the nucleus of the solitary tract (NTS). The human proglucagon gene is located on the long arm of chromosome 2. GLP-1 and -2 have 50% homology to glucagon, hence their names. Tissue-specific processing of proglucagon by PC2 and PC1/3 leads to the generation of glucagon in the pancreas and GLP-1 and -2, oxyntomodulin (OXM) and glicentin in the intestine, respectively (Fig. 1.2). Small quantities of GLP-1 have also been identified in the pancreas (due to the expression of PC1/3 in a minority of α cells), although the significance of this is not yet clear. Truncated GLP-1 peptides, GLP-1$_{7-36}$ and GLP-1$_{7-37}$ are biologically active with GLP-1$_{7-36}$ being the major circulatory form. In man, the majority of circulating GLP-1 is amidated, probably through the action of peptidyl-glycine α-amidating monooxygenase. The N-terminus of the peptide is essential for biological activity whereas the C-terminal is important for GLP-1 receptor binding. Soon after its discovery, the incretin effect of GLP-1 was quickly established in man.[6]

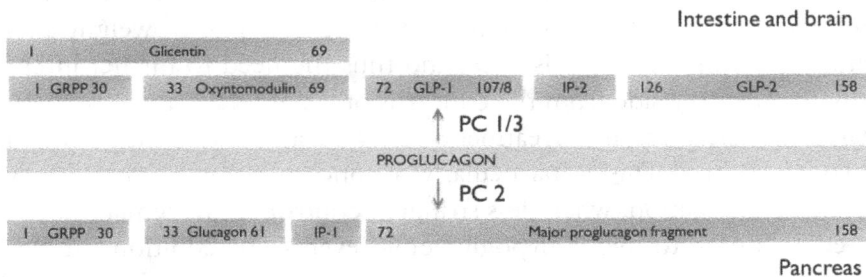

Figure 1.2. Differential post-translational processing of proglucagon in the pancreas, gut and brain. In the gut, glicentin-related polypeptide (GRPP), OXM, GLP-1, intervening peptide 2 (IP-2) and GLP-2 are formed. In the pancreas, GRPP, glucagon, intervening peptide 1 (IP-1) and major proglucagon fragment (MPGF) are formed.

1.4. Review of the Field

Diabetes affects about 347 million people worldwide, less than half of whom are adequately controlled (for more information see the International Diabetes Federation website at http://www.idf.org). Insulin resistance, particularly of the liver and skeletal muscle, underlies the pathogenesis of type 2 diabetes (T2D). Pancreatic β cells hypersecrete insulin in order to overcome this resistance and maintain euglycaemia. T2D is notoriously diagnosed late, by which time more than 80% of β cell function has often been lost. To diagnose T2D, post-prandial glucose measurement by an oral glucose tolerance test (OGTT) is considered the gold standard. More recently, measurement of glycated haemoglobin (HbA1c) of greater than 48 mmol/mol has been considered sufficient for diagnosis. However, in situations where there has been a rapid deterioration in glucose control (for example in pregnancy, steroid use or acute pancreatitis), HbA1c is not a reliable method to diagnose diabetes. Whilst fasting blood glucoses are often measured (reliable and cost-effective) these may give misleadingly normal results, as these are not affected until there is significant β cell loss.

There are already a number of treatment options for people with T2D; however, aside from metformin, many anti-hyperglycaemia treatments (sulfonylureas, thiazolidinediones, metaglinides and insulin) cause weight gain. There is often a vicious cycle of weight gain and increasing insulin resistance, and thus the need to further intensify treatment. Aside from the concerns of weight gain, these particular anti-hyperglycaemia treatments are also associated with risks of hypoglycaemia. This is particularly a concern amongst the elderly diabetic population, where less stringent control of glycaemia is tolerated in order to avoid hypoglycaemic events. In addition, in this elderly population insulin dosing is often problematic and there may be difficulties with insulin administration, visual acuity or memory. Furthermore, people with diabetes are frequently reluctant to initiate insulin therapy partly because of the stigma attached, especially amongst certain ethnic groups. Thus, there is a need for treatments for diabetes which are not associated with the risks of hypoglycaemia or the side effects of weight gain and, which are not stigmatised. This is where incretin therapy plays an important role.

The incretin effect is thought to be reduced in T2D, largely through diminished actions on the β cell of both GLP-1 (which are partial) and GIP (which are more substantial), with less evidence for a decrease in the circulating levels of either peptide. There are conflicting data on the secretion and activity of GLP-1 in T2D, with some studies demonstrating that GLP-1 levels are maintained and others showing a reduction. This is discussed in Chapter 7. Given the loss of GIP efficacy in T2D, GIP analogues have not been developed for use in diabetes treatment. By contrast, GLP-1 receptor agonists and analogues are effective agents in T2D. The latter have been available for clinical use since 2005 in the US and 2006 in the UK.

1.5. GIP and GLP-1 Release

GIP and GLP-1 are released from the intestine following food intake (fats, proteins and carbohydrates). Plasma levels of both GIP and GLP-1 are low in the fasted state and rise within minutes of a meal. The fasting plasma concentration of GLP-1 is 5–10 pmol/L and this can treble following food intake. GIP circulates in tenfold higher concentrations compared to GLP-1; however, GLP-1 is much more potent than GIP. The incretin effect of these hormones is additive. Importantly, GLP-1 and GIP are unstable in the bloodstream and rapidly degraded, with half-lives of 1–2 minutes and 7 minutes, respectively.

GIP is released from entero-endocrine K cells in the duodenum, whereas GLP-1 is released mainly from entero-endocrine L cells with increasing concentrations located distally in the large intestine and rectum. The release of GLP-1 occurs extremely rapidly following food intake, more rapidly than the time taken for direct stimulation of distal GLP-1 containing cells. Thus it was thought likely that a proximal-distal connection exists, achieved either hormonally or via the enteric nervous system. GLP-1 secretion displays a biphasic profile with an initial peak of release at 30 minutes followed by a second phase several hours later. More sophisticated techniques localising

GLP-1-containing cells have now demonstrated their presence more proximally in the gut.[7] In fact, the distinction between K and L cells is now less clearly defined. The mechanisms controlling hormone release and the distinction between these cell types are described in more detail in Chapter 2.

1.6. GIP and GLP-1 Receptors

The actions of both GIP and GLP-1 are mediated by G-protein-coupled receptors. Despite their structural homology to glucagon, GLP-1 and GLP-2 ligand binding is specific at their respective receptors; glucagon binds to the GLP-1 receptor with 100 times lower affinity than GLP-1. Receptor binding is coupled to adenylyl cyclase activation, cAMP formation and also — at least in some of the target cells — increased intracellular Ca^{2+}. Due to the paucity of reliable antibodies against these receptors, there has been much controversy over receptor localisation. Immunohistochemistry is notoriously unreliable and there is often discordance between receptor localisation using immunohistochemistry compared to receptor ligand binding studies and RNA analysis by polymerase chain reaction. Receptor localisation on target cells, and downstream signalling pathways, are described more fully in Chapters 3–5.

1.7. Clearance of Incretins

GIP and GLP-1 are rapidly inactivated by N-terminal cleavage at the alanine at position 2 by dipeptidyl peptidase IV (DPP-IV), also known as T cell antigen CD26. DPP-IV degradation occurs as GIP and GLP-1 encounter DPP-IV-impregnated blood vessels draining the intestinal mucosa. DPP-IV is also present in the kidney, intestinal brush-border, and hepatocytes. GIP_{1-42} is cleaved to inactive GIP_{3-42}, and GLP-1 to inactive $GLP-1_{9-37}$ or $GLP-1_{9-36}$. Neutral endopeptidase 24.11 also degrades GLP-1. Resulting degradation fragments are then cleared by the kidney. Incretin clearance is extremely rapid, and thus it is not clear if the effect on the pancreas is direct or indirect due to paracrine effects of the hormones and the enteric nervous system.

Importantly, and of relevance to the action of agents that target this enzyme, DPP-IV has a wide range of other substrates including the pancreatic polypeptide family, neuropeptide Y (NPY) and peptide YY (PYY), and a range of chemokines involved in immune regulation.

1.8. Functions of GLP-1

1.8.1. *GLP-1 and Glucose Homeostasis*

The actions of GLP-1 on glucose homeostasis are via the effects on the α cell and inhibition of glucagon secretion (described in Chapter 4), β cell and release of insulin (Chapter 3) and in the brain (Chapter 5). In addition, GLP-1 inhibits hepatic glucose production although, and importantly, it is not clear if hepatocytes express the GLP-1 receptor. Therefore the effect of GLP-1 on the liver may be direct or indirect, acting through other hormones (including insulin) or the central nervous system (CNS).

GIP and GLP-1 both stimulate glucose-dependent insulin secretion. However, GLP-1 has additional actions in the β cell, including the stimulation of insulin synthesis and (at least in some species) islet proliferation. Notably, the transcription factor pancreas duodenum homeobox 1 (Pdx-1), is a target of GLP-1 and implicated in the effects on insulin gene expression and proliferation in β cells. Following partial pancreatectomy in the rat, GLP-1 promotes islet expansion through proliferative and anti-apoptotic pathways. Moreover, GLP-1 has been shown to reduce pro-apoptotic signalling pathways (e.g. caspase-3) and enhance anti-apoptotic pathways (e.g. Bcl-2). In isolated human islets, GLP-1 has also been shown to have anti-apoptotic effects. However, it is not yet clear whether GLP-1 exerts this same control of β cell growth in man.

1.8.2. *GLP-1 and Appetite*

GLP-1 is considered a satiety signal implicated in the short-term regulation of feeding behaviour. GLP-1 receptors and GLP-1-expressing neurons are both located in areas of the brain associated with food intake, notably the ventromedial hypothalamus and the hind-brain. Correspondingly, GLP-1 administration leads to an acute reduction in food intake and a chronic reduction in body weight. GLP-1 is also associated with taste aversion, via stimulation of alternate neural pathways. This property may contribute to the anorectic effects of the peptide.

GLP-1 also regulates food transit through the gastrointestinal tract. Thus, following food ingestion, GLP-1 release inhibits upper gastrointestinal motility and slows gastric emptying, i.e. GLP-1 mediates the ileal break (important for nutrient absorption). This function of GLP-1 appears to be mediated by the vagus nerve as it is lost in vagal nerve ablation. GLP-1 also inhibits gastric acid secretion and pancreatic exocrine function.

Finally, the effects of GLP-1 are not limited to glucose regulation, metabolism and appetite. Although the contributions of these effects to the action of the incretin are debated (and some may be indirect), evidence also exists that GLP-1 acts on skeletal muscle, adipose tissue, bone, the heart and the brain, exerting neuroprotective effects in the latter case. In adipocytes, GLP-1 stimulates glucose uptake, lipogenesis and lipolysis. In brown adipose tissue (BAT), GLP-1 has an indirect effect via the CNS and increases thermogenesis.

1.8.3. *GLP-1 and the Thyroid and Bone*

GLP-1 receptor null mice are osteopenic; however, GLP-1 receptors have not been identified in bone, suggesting that the actions of the hormone on bone may be indirect. GLP-1 receptors are expressed on rodent thyroid C cells, which secrete calcitonin (a hormone which inhibits bone resorption). Thus it is possible that GLP-1 stimulates calcitonin secretion, which prevents bone resorption. This also has implications on the side effects of GLP-1 agonists seen in rodents (discussed in Chapter 8).

1.9. Functions of GIP

As well as serving as an incretin, GIP has been shown to exert anti-apoptotic effects on pancreatic β cells. However, and in contrast to

GLP-1, GIP does not exert effects on gastric emptying or food intake. Instead, the predominant role for GIP appears to be in the regulation of postprandial glucose levels, with no action to control fasting glucose. Counter-intuitively, GIP also stimulates glucagon secretion (see Chapter 4). Finally, GIP also exerts effects on white adipose tissue, where it increases lipid uptake and expansion of adipose depots and promotes weight gain.

1.10. Clinical Applications of the Incretin Hormones

1.10.1. *GLP-1-Based Therapies Based on Exendin-4*

GLP-1 administration reduces both fasting and postprandial glucose levels without causing hypoglycaemia. However, and as discussed in Section 1.7, degradation of GLP-1 by DPP-IV is extremely rapid. Thus, initially the only way to administer GLP-1 was by continuous intravenous infusion. The long-awaited therapeutic potential of incretins was only realised following the discovery of a high affinity GLP-1 agonist, exendin-4 (Ex4). This is a compound derived from the venom of the Gila monster lizard, *Heloderma suspectum*, and is 53% homologous to GLP-1. Importantly, glycine replaces alanine at position 2, protecting the peptide from DPP-IV-catalysed degradation. In November 2006, the first GLP-1 receptor agonist, exenatide, was approved in Europe, as a twice daily injectable. Shortly afterwards liraglutide (NN2211) was developed, injected once daily. Liraglutide has a fatty acyl tail which allows the molecule to associate with albumin and reduces renal elimination. A long-acting exenatide analogue, exenatide LA, (administered by weekly injection) was approved in 2011. In the latter preparation, exenatide is encased in a polylactide-glycolide microsphere suspension, greatly slowing metabolism of the peptide.

Clinical trials demonstrate that Ex4 is effective in lowering blood glucose, reducing HbA1c and causing weight loss. These effects are also seen in patients receiving concomitant metformin and sulphonylureas. However, it should be noted that the concomitant use of sulfonylureas and incretin therapy leads to the loss of the glucose-dependence of incretin action, and this can result in hypoglycaemia.

Table 1.1.	GLP-1 agonists in current use and in development.

Drug	Structure	Dosing regime
Exenetide (Byetta) AstraZeneca	Based on the structure of exendin-4.	Initiate at 5 mcg sc BD for 1 month, 60 minutes before breakfast and dinner. Increase to 10 mcg sc BD after 1 month.
Exenetide LAR (Bydureon)	Based on the structure of exendin-4.	2 mg sc weekly.
Lixisenatide (Lyxumia)	Based on the structure of exendin-4 with C-terminal modification.	10 mcg sc OD for 14 days. Increase to 20 mcg sc OD.
Albiglutide (Tanzeum) GSK	Tandem GLP-1 dimer fused to albumin.	Initiate at 30 mg once weekly. Dosing can be titrated up to 50 mg weekly.
Liraglutide (Victoza) Novo Nordisk	C16-acyl group attached to Lys via a glutamate linker.	Initiate at 0.6 mg sc OD for 1 week, and then increase to 1.2 mg sc OD. Available at 1.8 mg OD (but not recommended by NICE).
Dulaglutide (Trulicity) Eli Lilly	GLP-1 analogue linked to Fc of IgG4.	0.75 mg sc weekly; can increase to 1.5 mg weekly.

1.10.2. *DPP-IV Antagonists*

DPP-IV antagonists have also been used to prolong the half-life of GLP-1. Sitagliptin was the first clinically approved DPP-IV inhibitor. DPP-IV inhibitors have significant anti-diabetic effects; however, in contrast to GLP-1 agonists, they are weight neutral. The loss of the beneficial effects on weight may be due to the effects of DPP-IV on the anorectic hormone, PYY. The long-term side effects of DPP-IV inhibitors have not yet been determined; however, so far the main risks are a slightly increased risk of urinary tract infection, headache and nasopharyngitis. In general, the DPP-IV inhibitors have a good safety profile; however, they do not have a huge impact on glucose amelioration.

1.10.3. *Side Effects and Contra-Indications of Incretin Therapy*

The main side effects of incretin therapy are gastrointestinal, including nausea, vomiting, and diarrhoea. Often these side effects can be reduced by altering the timing of the drug with relation to the mealtime. The risks of pancreatitis and the potential of these drugs to cause tumorigenesis are discussed further in Chapter 8. Patients who have a history of gallstones, high alcohol intake or high triglyceride levels should not be started on incretin therapy. Patients with a personal or family history of medullary thyroid cancer or multiple endocrine neoplasia 2 (MEN2) should not be started on incretin therapy.

1.11. Stepwise Approach in Treatment of T2D

The target HbA1c in people with T2D is 6.5% or 48 mmol/mol (to approximately convert mmol/mol to percentage, add 24 and divide by 11). It is advised that glucose levels and HbA1c are monitored regularly every two to six months until the patient is stable on unchanging therapy. Once levels are stable, monitoring can be reduced to every six months. The following is a stepwise approach to T2D treatment advocated by the National Institute of Health and Care Excellence (NICE guideline 87, 2011).

1. If HbA1c is > 6.5% despite lifestyle measures, then start metformin. Sulphonylureas can be considered if (1) the patient is not overweight, (2) metformin is contraindicated (for example in renal failure) or (3) a rapid response is required due to the presence of hyperglycaemic symptoms.
2. If HbA1c is still > 6.5%, then a sulfonylurea can be added. At this stage a DPP-IV inhibitor or thiazolidinedione can be substituted if there are concerns regarding hypoglycaemia.
3. Current guidelines advise adding insulin if the HbA1c is > 7.5%. However, as discussed in Section 1.4, many people (patients and doctors) are reluctant to initiate insulin. Therefore, at this stage a DPP-IV inhibitor such as sitagliptin can be added. This can be continued if there is a reduction in HbA1c of > 0.5 in 6 months.

4. If the BMI > 35 (or < 35 with significant comorbidities), then a
   GLP-1 agonist, such as exenatide or liraglutide, can be added. This
   can be continued if there is a reduction in HbA1c of greater than
   1% or weight loss of more than 3% in 6 months. Of note, the combination of GLP-1 agonists and sulphonylureas negates the
   glucose dependent properties of the incretins and leads to a risk of
   hypoglycaemia. In addition, the concomitant use of DPP-IV
   inhibitors and GLP-1 agonists is not advised, as this increases the
   risk of pancreatitis.

1.12. Which Analogue is Best?

In 2009, a trial comparing exenatide and liraglutide (LEAD-6) in
patients already on metformin and or sulphonylureas demonstrated
that both reduced glucose levels, triglycerides, and weight (3 kg over
6 months), with a slight superiority of liraglutide.[8]

1.13. Incretin Plus Insulin

In the UK, NICE guidelines do not recommend the use of incretin
therapy in combination with insulin. However, audits of UK patient
data demonstrate that many patients already use exenatide as an add-
on treatment to a long-acting insulin. These patients do better than
those already on long-acting insulin who exchange this for an incretin
based therapy. In the US and Europe, exenatide has been licensed to
be used with basal insulin. Trials looking at the effectiveness of this
combination have shown positive effects both on glycaemic control
and on weight.

1.14. GLP-1 and the Myocardium

Cardiovascular disease is the leading cause of death worldwide and
T2D and obesity increase the risk of atherosclerosis and concomitant
ischaemic heart disease. GLP-1 agonists have been said to have a cardioprotective role and to reduce heart rate and blood pressure.
GLP-1 therefore may improve myocardial function and cardiac

output following myocardial injury. Interestingly, GLP-1_{7-36} (as well as the degradation product GLP-1_{9-36}) exerts beneficial cardiac effects. On the other hand, recent data using more specific antibodies suggest that GLP-1 receptors (GLP-1Rs) are concentrated in atrial, rather than ventricular myocytes, hinting that in this case improvements in cardiac performance after administration of GLP-1 agonists or stabilisers may be at least in part indirect.

1.15. GLP-1 Agonists and the Liver

T2D and obesity, and the combination of these two, are associated with the development of non-alcoholic steatosis (NASH), which is part of the spectrum of non-alcoholic fatty liver disease (NAFLD). NASH is often not associated with any signs or symptoms but rather causes elevations in aminotransferases. NASH is rapidly becoming the most common cause of chronic liver disease. Whilst it is often mild in nature, it has the potential to progress to cirrhosis and liver failure. GLP-1 agonists have been shown to reduce levels of steatosis in the liver. Currently, it is not clear if this is caused by a direct effect (as previously mentioned the presence of GLP-1R in the liver is not yet firmly established) or if this is due to weight loss caused by the agonists.

1.16. Incretin Use in Type 1 Diabetes

Incretin therapy clearly has a role where there are functioning β cells to act upon. However, the utility of incretins in type 1 diabetes has been queried. In studies examining the effects of liraglutide or exenatide LAR in patients with type 1 diabetes ($n = 14$, $n = 11$, respectively), glucose levels dropped and insulin requirements decreased within one week. This effectiveness of incretin therapy in type 1 diabetes may signify the presence of a few functioning β cells, or equally may be attributed to the actions of suppressing glucagon release from α cells. The presence of functioning β cells can be estimated by measuring glucagon stimulated C-peptide levels. Further trials of GLP-1 agonists in both C-peptide-positive and C-peptide-negative patients with type 1 diabetes have demonstrated a reduction in the total daily insulin dose as well as the HbA1c. However, GLP-1 agonist treatment did not increase C-peptide levels. Currently, incretin therapy is not licensed for patients with type 1 diabetes.

1.17. Key Experimental Approaches

Progress in peptide chemistry and the development of assays, notably the radioimmunoassay (RIA) in the 1960s, led to the acceleration of research surrounding GLP-1. In order to investigate incretins it is important that we have the tools to accurately measure them and understand the results.

1.17.1. *GLP-1 Measurement in Plasma*

GLP-1 levels vary with food intake; thus it is prudent to measure either fasting levels of GLP-1 or levels after a fixed meal. It has also been shown that gut hormone levels vary with exercise and the previous evening's meal. Thus, in a study it is sensible to standardise the previous evening's meal, and to dictate that the subject uses the same method of transport to attend the study and does not exercise the evening prior to the study.

It is also established that DPP-IV rapidly degrades GLP-1 (see above). Therefore, in order to measure active GLP-1, DPP-IV inhibitors should be added to the test tube. The synthetic tripeptide Ile-pro-ile, otherwise known as Diprotin A, is a classic DPP-IV inhibitor and cleverly provides an excess of substrate which overwhelms the enzymes' capacity to cleave the position-two alanine in GLP-1. In addition, other degradative enzymes exist in plasma, so it is useful to add a non-specific protease inhibitor to the sample, such as aprotinin, (trasylol) 1000–5000 kallikrein units per ml of blood. In 2012 trasylol was banned by the FDA for use for medicinal purposes. As a result it has become more difficult to obtain for use in the lab. It is not clear if it is essential to add this as we were unable to find comparative studies looking at the effects of adding or omitting trasylol to samples. Other enzyme inhibitors include phenyl methane sulfonyl fluoride (PMSF), effective concentration 0.1–1 mM.

1.17.1.1. *Protocol*

(1) Collect the blood sample into a green top tube containing sodium heparin with DPP-IV inhibitor, DpA (0.1 mmol/L) and aprotinin (aprotinin concentrate 20,000 KIU; add 50 μl per mL plasma or blood to give a final concentration of 1000 KIU per mL).

(2) Invert the tube several times and keep on ice until centrifugation at 3000 g for 15 minutes. Remove the plasma using a Pasteur pipette and store aliquots in 1.5 mL Eppendorf tubes. Freeze upright and store at −80°C until assayed. Note that repeat freeze-thaw cycles will result in peptide degradation.

(3) Active levels or total GLP-1 levels can be measured. We use an in-house RIA to measure total GLP-1 levels and an enzyme-linked immunosorbent assay (ELISA) to measure active GLP-1 (e.g. Millipore, formally Linco Research).

1.17.2. *GLP-1 Levels in Tissue*

Occasionally, you may need to measure GLP-1 levels in tissue. GLP-1 is stable at 100°C whereas enzymes are not. Thus it is possible to extract and preserve GLP-1 by boiling tissue in acid at 100°C for 15 minutes. As GLP-1 levels vary throughout the gut and the density of L cells is region specific, it is important to measure and record the area where the tissue was sampled, e.g. 50 cm from the pylorus.

1.17.2.1. *Protocol*

(1) Prepare a 0.5M solution of acetic acid (10 mL distilled water and 300 μL glacial acetic acid).

(2) Weigh an Eppendorf and add 1 mL of 0.5M acetic acid to the Eppendorf.

(3) Boil the tube for 10 minutes so that it reaches 100°C. It may be necessary to use a pressure cooker.

(4) Add a small piece of fresh tissue to the tube (about 1 mm^3) and reweigh.
(5) Boil for 15 minutes.
(6) Remove, cool tube and reweigh.
(7) The hormone will have dispersed from the tissue, which will not have completely dissolved, and be present in the acetic acid.
(8) Store at −20°C until assay.
(9) Use two standard curves and to one add 0.5M acetic acid to determine if the assay is affected by the acetic acid. If it is, dilute the samples until there is minimal interference by the acid.
(10) Express the hormone in relation to the wet weight of the tissue e.g. pmol/g wet weight.

1.17.3. *Staining Tissues for GLP-1: Immunohistochemistry*

Staining tissues for GLP-1 can cause enormous problems due to issues with antibody sensitivity. Thus, it is essential to have positive and negative controls and, if possible, to use antibodies that have been used in published and peer-reviewed papers. The gold-standard negative control is a tissue that does not contain the antigen. If these tissues are not available then it is possible to pre-adsorb the antiserum against the peptide the antibody was raised against (however, this does not protect against cross reaction of the antibody). Omission controls, where the primary antibody is left out, demonstrate specificity of the secondary antibody alone and do not give additional information about the primary antibody. In general, frozen tissues are easier to stain and are less likely to require antigen retrieval steps, whereas paraffin-embedded tissues often require an antigen retrieval step. However, these give a higher clarity image.

1.18. Key Challenges/Gaps in the Field

1.18.1. *Clinical Gaps*

Much of what is known about incretin biology has been determined from animal models. However, there are significant differences between animal models and man. In particular, it has been difficult to investigate the *in vivo* effect of incretins on pancreatic survival and regeneration and much of what is known has been extrapolated from animal data or surmised from surrogate markers.

1.18.2. *Drug Delivery*

The harsh digestive environment makes it difficult to administer peptide hormones orally. Initial research into the incretin field was delayed by a lack of understanding of peptide degradation and the variable results obtained following oral administration of incretin extracts. A century later, administration of peptide drugs is still problematic, although various novel drug delivery solutions are being developed. Administration of GLP-1 is still by injection; however, longer acting analogues that can be administered weekly are now available.

1.18.3. *Interfering Antibodies*

Injection of peptide stimulates an immune response and antibodies may develop against the injected peptide. More is known about insulin antibodies; to date, the immune reactions are not severe and often only necessitate higher doses of insulin to overcome this interference. It is hypothetically possible that anaphylaxis develops against a peptide injection. However, this does not appear to be a problem in practice.

1.18.4. *When to Start GLP-1?*

Current NICE guidelines advocate the use of GLP-1 analogues as third-line agents in obese patients with T2D. However, the mechanism of action of incretins suggests that they are best used early on in T2D, prior to β cell failure. NICE guidelines try to balance cost and clinical efficacy and currently the cost of incretin therapy is higher than sulfonylureas or thiazolidinediones, hence its placement as a third-line agent.

1.18.5. *What are the Long-Term Consequences of Injected GLP-1?*

This will be discussed fully in Chapter 8 but to date the long term consequences of GLP-1 treatment are not clear. Concerns about thyroid and pancreatic cancer have been raised; however, it is not clear if there is a causal link. In reality, these conditions are so rare that most studies are insufficiently powered to be able to determine if these malignancies are associated with incretin use.

1.19. Conclusions

- The incretin effect is defined as the greater insulin release after an oral compared to an intravenous glucose load.
- GLP-1 and GIP both have incretin effects. However, in diabetes, β cells lose responsiveness to GIP so this has not been a clinically useful entity.
- In addition to being an incretin, GLP-1 has beneficial pleiotropic effects including: reduction of appetite, inducement of weight loss, neuroprotective effects and beneficial cardiac effects.
- Various GLP-1 receptor agonists and analogues have been developed. These are resistant to DPP-IV degradation and some have additions (such as a fatty acid tail or combination with albumin) to prevent renal clearance. DPP-IV inhibitors have also been successfully used to increase longevity of endogenous incretins.
- Since 2006, GLP-1 receptor agonists have been licenced for use in obese patients with diabetes and these have been a useful clinical adjunct and have been shown in trials to reduce HbA1c and body weight.
- GLP-1 may have a role in patients with T2D already on insulin, and possibly in type 1 diabetes.

References

1. Bayliss, W.M. and Starling, E.H. (1902). The mechanism of pancreatic secretion, *The Journal of Physiology*, **28**(5), 325–353.
2. La Barre, J. and Still, E.U. (2009). "III. Further Studies on the Effects of Secretin on the Blood Sugar", in *Studies on the Physiology of Secretin*, Laboratories of Physiology and Pharmacology of the University of Chicago, Chicago, IL, pp. 649–653.
3. Unger, R.H. and Eisentraut, A.M. (1969). Entero-insular axis, *Arch. Intern. Med.*, **123**(3), 261–266.
4. Brown, J.C. and Dryburgh, J.R. (1971). A gastric inhibitory polypeptide. II. The complete amino acid sequence, *Can. J. Biochem.*, **49**(8), 867–872.

5. Bell, G.I., Santerre, R.F. and Mullenbach, G.T. (1983). Hamster preproglucagon contains the sequence of glucagon and two related peptides, *Nature*, **302**(5910), 716–718.

6. Kreymann, B., Williams, G., Ghatei, M.A. and Bloom, S.R. (1987). Glucagon-like peptide-1 7–36: A physiological incretin in man, *Lancet*, **2**(8571), 1300–1304.

7. Hansen, C.F., Vrang, N., Sangild, P.T. and Jelsing, J. (2013). Novel insight into the distribution of L-cells in the rat intestinal tract, *Am. J. Transl. Res.*, **5**(3), 347–358.

8. Buse, J.B., Rosenstock, J., Sesti, G., Schmidt, W. E., Montanya, E., Brett, J.H., Zychma, M. and Blonde, L. (LEAD-6 Study Group) (2009). Liraglutide once a day versus exenatide twice a day for type 2 diabetes: A 26-week randomised, parallel-group, multinational, open-label trial (LEAD-6), *Lancet*, **374**(9683), 39–47.

Chapter 2

Synthesis and Secretion
of Incretins from the Gut

A.E. Adriaenssens, F. Reimann and F. Gribble

*MRC Metabolic Diseases Unit, Institute of Metabolic Science,
University of Cambridge*

2.1. Introduction

In addition to the absorption of nutrients from digested food, one of
the primary roles of the intestine is to act as a dynamic sensory organ.
Gastrointestinal motility and mucosal transport need to be tuned to
the availability of food within the gut lumen, but the intestine also
sends signals to other organs, thus playing an integral part in activating regulatory mechanisms employed to cope with the body's chang-
ing nutritional status. Entero-endocrine cells, secreting around twenty
identified hormones, play an important part in this communication.

Arguably some of the most therapeutically enticing signals released
from the gut are the incretin hormones, glucagon-like peptide-1 (GLP-1)
and glucose-dependent insulinotropic polypeptide (GIP), which modulate the endocrine pancreas and thus affect the fate of absorbed glucose.
Following the success in the treatment of hyperglycaemia of synthetic
GLP-1 mimetics and dipeptidyl peptidase-IV (DPP-IV) inhibitors,
which prolong incretin action, there is strong interest in how the
endogenous incretin axis might be stimulated as a therapeutic target for

metabolic disorders. The approximately 80% remission rate of diabetes after bariatric surgery procedures such as Roux-en-Y gastric bypass (RYGB) is associated with robust increases in postprandial plasma GLP-1 responses, proving that there is a recruitable "reserve" pool of GLP-1 in patients with diabetes. Learning more about the physiological regulation of incretin-releasing cells will therefore be crucial to harness the incretin axis in the treatment of metabolic diseases.

The aim of this chapter is to describe what is currently known about cell signalling pathways that underlie direct nutrient-mediated regulation of incretin-releasing cells. We will also outline key methodologies and describe transgenic mouse lines used to study incretin-secreting cells at the single-cell level. Gaps in our understanding of regulatory pathways as well as methodological challenges that this field faces will be discussed.

2.2. Review of the Field

Though entero-endocrine cells comprise less than one percent of the total gastrointestinal epithelial cell population, it is now recognised that they collectively make up the body's largest endocrine organ. Arguably, however, they remain one of the least well-understood branches of the endocrine system. GIP and GLP-1 are respectively secreted from so-called K and L cells, which are found scattered throughout the gastrointestinal epithelium. The highest density of K cells is found in the duodenum, while the highest density of L cells is found in the ileum and colon. An early rise in postprandial plasma GIP and GLP-1 levels begins within minutes of food ingestion, and a prolonged phase of secretion lasts for a further 1–3 h, depending on the macronutrient composition of the meal. It has been argued that because the early phase of secretion happens rapidly, neural or hormonal signals must play a role in initiating GLP-1 secretion from the distal L cell population. Recent evidence, however, favours the alternative view that direct sensing of luminal contents by proximal L cells is sufficient to account for the early rise of GLP-1. Thus, the onset, peak and duration of glucose-stimulated GLP-1 release are in line with the time course of glucose arriving at different regions of the small intestine, and patients that have undergone RYGB exhibit elevated post-prandial GLP-1 levels, most likely due to higher concentrations of nutrients reaching segments of the intestine that are more densely populated with L cells.

A key feature of L and K cells is that they are polarised, open-type entero-endocrine cells, meaning that their apical surface is lined with microvilli that protrude into the gut lumen. This allows L and K cells to directly sense passing luminal nutrients and release GLP-1- or GIP-containing secretory granules from their broader basolateral surface. Indeed, L and K cells release their respective incretin hormones in response to all three classes of macronutrients: carbohydrate, protein, and fat. This nutrient-mediated regulation of L and K cells makes these cells important players in neural and endocrine pathways that link nutritional status with glucose homeostasis.

2.3. Differential Nutrient Sensing and Novel Tools

As L and K cells constitute very rare cell types and are not readily distinguishable from other epithelial cells during live-cell light microscopy, knowledge of the signalling pathways regulating nutrient-stimulated incretin release used to be derived from ingestion studies in humans and animals, and perfusion studies in whole segments of intestine. Some molecular characterisation was also possible in *in vitro* models, e.g. model cell lines such as GLUTag and STC-1 and primary cultures of fetal rat intestinal epithelium. Experiments exploring different nutrient stimulus–secretion coupling mechanisms in L and K cells at the single cell level have, however, been greatly aided by the development of transgenic mouse strains that allow the unambiguous identification of L and K cells through cell-specific expression of fluorescent proteins such as Venus (a derivative of yellow fluorescent protein (YFP)). Venus is targeted to a specific entero-endocrine cell population by harnessing the promoter of one of the cell's hormonal products, either to drive the expression of the fluorescent protein directly, or to drive it indirectly via Cre recombinase.

Mice with fluorescently labelled entero-endocrine cells have enabled fluorescence-assisted cell sorting (FACS) of primary L and K cells, resulting in the characterisation of the transcriptome of these cells. Whilst FACS-sorted cells, at least in our hands, did not show robust hormone secretion in response to nutrients, the parallel development of mixed

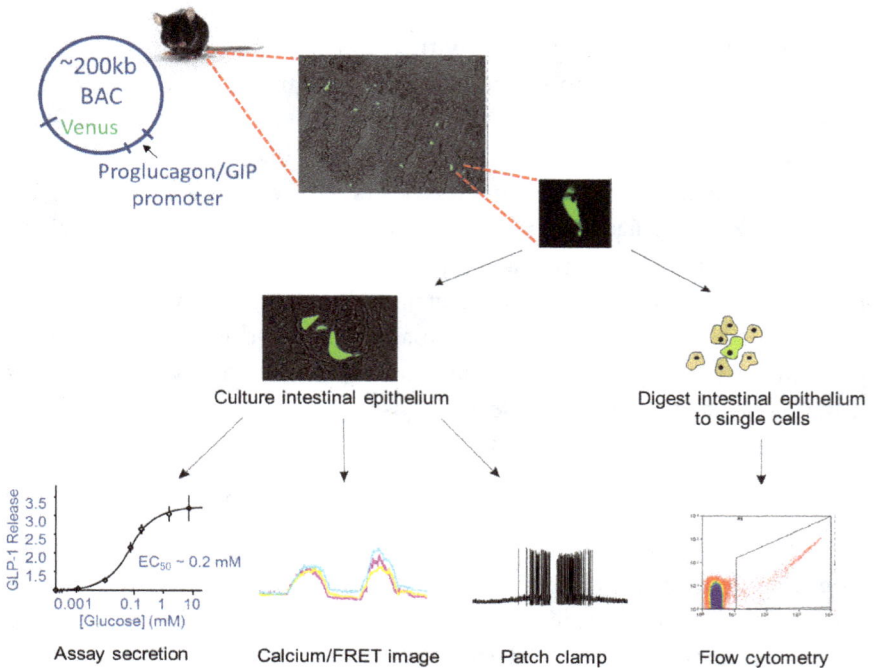

Figure 2.1. Transgenic mice are used in investigating nutrient detection in incretin cells. Intestinal epithelium from transgenic mice expressing fluorescent proteins under the control of either the proglucagon or GIP promoter is used to provide a means of examining regulatory mechanisms controlling incretin release at the single cell level. Crypts can be isolated from the epithelium and cultured to allow for electrophysiological characterisation and functional imaging using calcium indicators or fluorescence resonance energy transfer (FRET)-based probes. Bulk secretion assays can also be performed from cultured epithelium to examine the effect of various nutritional regulators on incretin release. The intestinal epithelium can also be digested to single cells to facilitate the purification of L and K cells via FACS. These isolated incretin cell populations can be used for gene expression analysis for the identification of novel therapeutic targets.

primary cultures of adult murine intestinal epithelium allowed *in vitro* screening of secretory stimuli. The fluorescent tag of the incretin-secreting cells enables cell identification, and can be used in parallel with single-cell techniques, including live-cell imaging and electro-physiological patch clamping, to monitor how the cells respond to different stimuli (Fig. 2.1). The mouse models expressing Cre recombinase

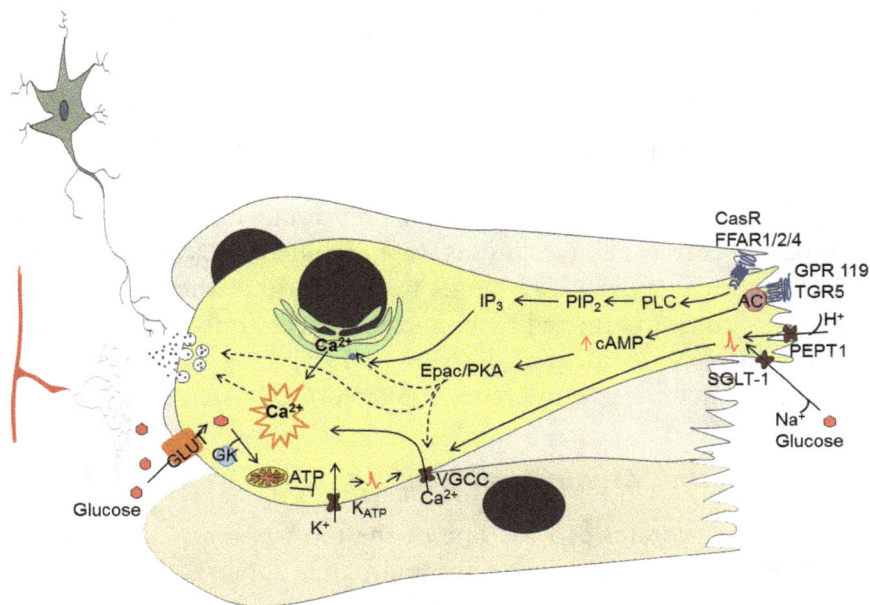

Figure 2.2.   Nutrient sensing in incretin-releasing cells. Glucose sensing proceeds through the electrogenic SGLT-1 transporter, giving rise to cell depolarisation. Glucose metabolism following GLUT-mediated uptake also contributes to L and K cell depolarisation via the closure of K_{ATP} channels. Cation-coupled amino acid or peptide (e.g. PEPT1) uptake also provides a depolarising stimulus. Membrane depolarisation activates VGCCs (voltage-gated calcium channels), stimulating Ca^{2+} influx and secretory granule release. L and K cells express a range of GPCRs, through which they detect the presence of fatty acids, bile acids and oligopeptides. G_s-coupled receptors (e.g. TGR5, GPR 119) elevate cAMP, activating PKA and Epac2, which have downstream effects on VGCC activity, Ca^{2+} release from intracellular stores, and secretory vesicle priming. G_q-coupled receptors (e.g. CasR, FFAR1/2/4) stimulate PLC and the release of Ca^{2+} from intracellular stores.

in a defined entero-endocrine cell population further allow genetic manipulation, such as cell-specific knockout of suspected key nutrient sensors after crossing with floxed alleles, or the cell-specific expression of a growing number of fluorescent sensors for monitoring of intracellular second messengers. Using this armoury of transgenic technology in combination with immortalised model cell lines, we have begun to dissect the electrophysiological characteristics and cell-signalling mechanisms that underlie L and K cell activity (Fig. 2.2).

2.3.1. *Incretin-Secreting Cells are Electrically Excitable*

Whole-cell patch clamping revealed that both murine model cell lines, STC-1 and GLUTag, are capable of firing action potentials. The underlying voltage-gated currents were characterised in detail in the GLUTag cell line and included voltage-gated sodium (Na_v) and calcium (Ca_v) currents, with the latter being dominated by L-type and N-type Ca_v current. Similar results were obtained in L cells in primary colonic cultures from GLU-Venus mice, although the calcium currents seem to be dominated by L- and P/Q-type. Importantly, blockage of either Na_v with tetrodotoxin or L-type Ca_v with nifedipine reduced nutrient (e.g. glutamine)-triggered GLP-1 secretion.

2.3.2. *Incretin Carbohydrate Sensing*

Simple carbohydrates provide one of the most potent secretagogues for incretin release, but are effective only when applied from the luminal side of the gut. Signalling mechanisms that may contribute to glucose sensing in L and K cells include the closure of ATP-sensitive K^+ channels (K_{ATP} channels) and the electrogenic activity of Na^+ glucose co-transporters (SGLTs). Other mechanisms proposed include the activation of gastducin-coupled sweet taste receptors (Tas1r2/3 heterodimers), although we were unable to stimulate incretin secretion in primary cultures with artificial sweeteners targeting these receptors, and mRNA expression levels for Tas1R-subunits were at or below the detection level by RT-PCR (reverse transcription polymerase chain reaction) in FACS-sorted K and L cells.

2.3.3. *Glucose Uptake Mechanisms*

2.3.3.1. *Facilitative hexose transport*

Facilitative hexose transport is mediated by the GLUT family of transporters. GLUTs are integral membrane proteins with mutually-exclusive glucose binding sites on their cytoplasmic and exoplasmic faces. Once glucose binds either the cytoplasmic or the exoplasmic binding site, a conformational change takes place to carry the glucose molecule from one side of the plasma membrane to the other. GLUT1, GLUT2 and, GLUT5 are known to be expressed in the intestine.

GLUT1 is a high-affinity (K_m = 3 mM) glucose transporter that is widely expressed throughout the body. GLUT2 has a low affinity (K_m = 17 mM) but high capacity. Principally found in the liver, pancreatic islets, brain, kidney, and intestine, GLUT2 has been implicated in glucose-sensing mechanisms that control feeding, energy expenditure, and counter-regulation during hypoglycaemia. In intestinal epithelial cells, GLUT2 expression is limited to the basolateral surface, and plays the major role in transporting glucose taken up from the intestinal lumen into the bloodstream. Groups have speculated that in the presence of high glucose concentrations, GLUT2 translocates to the apical surface of intestinal epithelial cells. However, the use of supraphysiological concentrations of glucose in these studies brings the relevance of a putative role for GLUT2 at the apical surface into question. GLUT5 is the principal fructose transporter throughout the body, though it is not involved in the transport of glucose. Importantly, the expression of GLUT transporters in the brush border is regulated by the concentration of circulating nutrients, and is altered in diabetes, suggesting that aberrations in carbohydrate uptake can contribute to the diseased state.

2.3.3.2. *Active glucose transport*

The primary mechanism of glucose absorption from the intestinal lumen proceeds uphill, against its concentration gradient. This active transport is enabled by a Na^+ gradient across the brush border membrane that is maintained by the basolaterally-located Na^+–K^+ ATPase. The apical membrane protein responsible for coupling glucose transport with an inward Na^+ current is SGLT-1. SGLT-1 is abundantly expressed in the intestine, where it is targeted to the brush border by its N-terminal domain. Its expression at the apical surface is positively regulated by glucose, a process thought to proceed via the activation of protein kinase A (PKA). In diabetes, the expression of SGLT-1 is upregulated, and Na^+/glucose co-transport activity is increased.

In addition to glucose, SGLT-1 is capable of transporting non-metabolisable glucose analogues, including 3-O-methyl-D-glucoside and α-methyl-D-glucopyranoside, a fact that is useful in distinguishing SGLT-1 versus metabolism-mediated glucose sensing. The electrogenic nature of SGLT-1-mediated glucose transport also sets it apart from GLUT/facilitative uptake, and is important to the role of SGLT-1 as a depolarising, excitatory glucose sensor.[1]

2.3.4. *Incretin Glucose Sensing*

2.3.4.1. *Closure of K_{ATP} channels*

Exploring the electrophysiology behind glucose-induced GLP-1 release in GLUTag cells revealed that L cells and pancreatic β cells may share a common glucose-sensing pathway. The canonical model of pancreatic β cell glucose sensing postulates that glucose is first transported into the cell via GLUT2 (in rodents) where it is phosphorylated by glucokinase. Subsequent glucose metabolism produces a rise in ATP and a corresponding drop in ADP. The increasing ATP and falling ADP concentrations close K_{ATP} channels, leading to membrane depolarisation. Membrane depolarisation initiates the opening of voltage-gated Ca^{2+} channels, and increased Ca^{2+} influx ultimately stimulates exocytosis.

We used perforated patch clamp experiments and secretion studies to show that glucose decreased GLUTag cell membrane conductance, an observation that was attributed to the closure of sulphonylurea-sensitive K_{ATP} channels.[2] FACS-purified populations of L and K cells, analysed by qRT-PCR (quantitative real time polymerase chain reaction), confirmed that both cell types express the K_{ATP} channel subunits SUR1 and Kir6.2, as well as glucokinase.[3,4] Secretion experiments confirmed the presence and function of K_{ATP} channels in glucose-stimulated GLP-1 and GIP release in primary intestinal epithelial cultures.

Despite the fact that K_{ATP} channels are present and functional in incretin-secreting cells, the therapeutic potential of this glucose-sensing pathway as a target for increasing endogenous incretin secretion is brought into question by clinical studies in humans showing that sulfonylurea treatment had no effect on incretin release in subjects challenged with an oral glucose tolerance test. Research focus therefore turned to identifying metabolism-independent mechanisms underlying glucose-stimulated incretin release.

2.3.5. *Na$^+$ Glucose Co-Transporters*

The presence of a metabolism-independent glucose-sensing mechanism in incretin cells is supported by experiments in perfused ileum preparations showing that the non-metabolisable sugars, 3-O-methylglucose and α-methylglucopyranoside (α-MG), induced GLP-1 and GIP secretion. Electrophysiological and secretion studies in GLUTag cells showed that the electrogenic activity of SGLT-1 accounted for Na$^+$-dependent GLP-1 secretion. It is now believed that both electrogenic sugar uptake and sugar metabolism contribute to the glucose sensitivity of incretin-releasing cells.[1] The EC$_{50}$ for glucose-mediated incretin release was found to be 0.2 mM, which closely mirrors the K_m for SGLT-1-mediated glucose transport. Definitive evidence for the integral role of SGLT-1 in mediating glucose-coupled incretin release came from experiments performed in SGLT-1 knockout mice. In these studies, SGLT-1 null mice exhibited a compromised first-phase incretin response to an oral glucose load.

Small molecules designed to inhibit SGLTs have paradoxically been shown to elicit significant increases in incretin release in response to oral glucose loads in humans and mice. Further studies showed that GLP-1 levels in SGLT-1 knockout mice were significantly elevated at delayed time points, compared to wild-type mice. As products of microbial fermentation are also potent secretagogues for incretin release, it has been postulated that the inhibition of glucose absorption following pharmaceutical or genetic blockade of SGLT-1 results in increased delivery of glucose to distal regions of the gut where microbes ferment the sugar into short chain fatty acids (SCFA), thereby stimulating L cells and increasing GLP-1 release. Alternatively, the resultant "dumping" of glucose into L-cell-rich distal regions in situations of compromised SGLT-1 activity could stimulate GLP-1 release via metabolism-dependent pathways. Investigations into SGLT-1-mediated regulation of incretin cells would benefit from a more targeted deletion of SGLT-1 solely in incretin cells.

2.3.6. *Lipid Sensing in Incretin-Secreting Cells*

Like carbohydrates, triglycerides are effective stimuli of incretin release, but only when applied from the luminal direction. Lipid-stimulated incretin release is dose-dependent and affected by the degree of fatty acid saturation, unsaturated fats being more potent GLP-1 secretagogues than saturated fats. The conversion of triglycerides to free fatty acids and 2-monoglyceride by pancreatic lipase is a critical step in fat-stimulated incretin release. G-protein coupled receptors (GPCRs) likely contribute to the stimulatory effects of fatty acids and lipid metabolites. Specifically, GPR119, GPR120 (FFAR4), GPR43 (FFAR2) and, GPR40 (FFAR1) have been found to be expressed in FACS-purified L and K cells. It is hoped that these GPCRs may offer new therapeutic targets for the augmentation of incretin release.

FFAR4 and FFAR1 are predominantly G_q-coupled receptors, activated by long-chain unsaturated fatty acids, which are coupled through the secondary messengers, inositol (1,4,5)-triphosphate (IP_3) and protein kinase C (PKC). The activation of IP_3 receptors leads to the release of Ca^{2+} from intracellular stores, which could ultimately stimulate vesicle exocytosis. The action of long-chain unsaturated fatty acids on GLP-1 and GIP secretion has also been attributed to activation of protein kinase C-ζ (PKC-ζ). FFAR2, by contrast, preferentially binds SCFA. Work in our laboratory confirmed the expression and functional activity of FFAR2 and its fellow SCFA sensor, FFAR3, in FACS-purified L cell populations, confirming previous immunohistochemistry results.[5] FFAR2 and FFAR3 knockout mice correspondingly exhibited impaired glucose tolerance compared to wild-type littermates. It is therefore plausible that these receptors contribute to a functional cross-talk between the gut microbiota and incretin cells that could be therapeutically relevant to improving glucose homeostasis in diabetic individuals.

Oleoylethanolamide (OEA) is an anorexogenic acylethanolamine, released from enterocytes in the intestinal brush border in response to ingested fats. It signals in part through GPR119, leading to elevating cAMP, which in turn potentiates glucose-mediated incretin secretion through the activation of PKA- and Epac2-dependent mechanisms.[6] It is hypothesised that the satiety-inducing properties of OEA could in part be mediated via incretin release. However, post-prandial concentrations of OEA are quite low, bringing into question whether OEA is a physiologically relevant intermediary of lipid-induced incretin release. 2-oleoylglycerol (2-OG), produced in the gut lumen by the hydrolysis of triacylglycerols, may provide a more plentiful lipid-derived agonist of GPR119.

Factors released to facilitate the processing of dietary fat also play key roles in incretin cell stimulation. Bile acid activation of the GPCR TGR5 triggers GLP-1 secretion in primary L cells[7] through a G_s-coupled pathway. TGR5 activation is also thought to be triggered by the increased delivery of bile salts into the jejunum of patients who have received RYGB surgery, contributing to the post-surgical increase in GLP-1 secretion seen in these patients.

2.3.7. *Incretin Protein Sensing*

Amino acids and oligopeptides are proven incretin secretatogues *in vivo, in vitro,* and in human studies. Some amino acids such as glutamine exhibit electrogenic nutrient transport capable of stimulating GLP-1 release. Whilst investigating the machinery necessary for glutamine-induced GLP-1 release, we found that glutamine-dependent L cell activation involved Na^+-coupled glutamine transport, suggesting that the cumulative action of brush border electrogenic nutrient transporters may trigger L cell excitability. In support of this idea, the sensing of oligopeptides in L cells was also partially dependent on ion flux, attributable to the proton-coupled electrogenic activity of PEPT1.[8]

GPCR signalling has also been implicated in L cell sensing of amino acids and oligopeptides. We found, for example, that oligopeptides triggered L cell Ca^{2+} transients and GLP-1 secretion that could be attributed to activation of the Ca^{2+} sensing receptor (CasR).[8] Contrary to previous reports, however, we were unable to link LPAR5 activity to GLP-1 secretion using primary cultures from knockout mouse strains,[8] leaving the role of this receptor in L cell nutrient sensing in question. In GLUTag cells, GPCR6A was demonstrated to mediate ornithine-stimulated GLP-1 release, but its role in primary tissue is unclear, as expression levels of this receptor are relatively low in primary L cells.[8]

2.4. Key Methods

2.4.1. *Transgenic Mouse Lines*

Real-time, single-cell analyses examining stimulus-secretion pathways in L and K cells were first enabled by transgenic mice that expressed the fluorescent protein, Venus, under the control of the glucagon or GIP promoter, respectively.[3,4] These two original glucagon and GIP transgenic mouse lines were created following the pro-nuclear injection of bacterial artificial chromosomes (BAC), engineered using the RedEt recombination method, into mouse ova. Further transgenic lines were developed using hormonal promoter sequences to drive the expression of Cre recombinase, allowing for the crossing in of ROSA26 floxed Cre reporter lines. These Cre reporter strains generally have a floxed "stop" sequence in front of the transgene driven by (a sometimes enhanced) ROSA26 promoter. In the presence of Cre recombinase, the stop sequence is irreversibly excised and the reporter sequence inverted in constructs in which it is inserted in reverse orientation, allowing the expression of the respective transgene. The models allow for the differentiation of L or K cells from neighbouring cells in mixed intestinal epithelial cultures, and for the introduction of genetically encoded calcium indicators (GECI), like GCaMP3.

We use several different crosses of Cre strains with ROSA26 floxed reporters to allow for the identification and purification of L and K cells, or for monitoring intracellular signalling factors to provide a read out of L or K cell activity. Key mouse lines are listed in Table 2.1.

2.4.2. *Probes Used for Measuring Signalling Factors*

In order to analyse the signalling pathways by which nutrients act on incretin cells, fluorescent probes have been employed that allow the visualisation of L or K cell excitation.

Table 2.1.   Trangenic mice used in studying L and K cells.

Mouse strain name	Cell type targeted	Transgene	Use
GLU-Venus	L cells	Venus driven by the gcg promoter.	FACS purification for gene expression analysis. Identification in mixed intestinal epithelial cultures for electrophysiology and calcium imaging following Fura-2AM loading.
GLU-Cre × ROSA26 GCaMP3	L cells	GCaMP3 restricted to L cells due to gcg promoter-driven cre.	Single cell, real-time calcium imaging. Avoids problems associated with poor loading of Fura-2AM, which works better in > 5-day-old cultures. Enables imaging of younger primary cultures.
GLU-Cre × ROSA26 tdRFP	L cells	tdRFP restricted to L cells due to gcg promoter-driven cre.	Identification in mixed intestinal epithelial cultures. Allows for the use of FRET-based probes with excitation wavelengths that would overlap with Venus. Can be crossed with ROSA26 GCaMP3 reporter lines, to enable easier identification of L cells (GCaMP3 fluorescence is dim at resting Ca^{2+} levels).
GIP-Venus	K cells	Venus driven by gip promoter.	FACS purification for gene expression analysis. Identification in mixed intestinal epithelial cultures for calcium imaging following Fura-2AM loading
GIP-Cre × ROSA26 GCaMP3	K cells	GCaMP3 restricted to K cells due to gip promoter-driven cre.	Single-cell, real-time calcium imaging. Avoids problems associated with poor loading of Fura-2AM.

(Continued)

Table 2.1.   (*Continued*)

Mouse strain name	Cell type targeted	Transgene	Use
GIP-Cre × ROSA26 tdRFP	K cells	tdRFP restricted to K cells due to gip promoter-driven cre	Identification in mixed intestinal epithelial cultures. Can be crossed with ROSA26 GCaMP3 reporter lines for easier identification of K cells.

2.4.2.1. *Calcium indicators*

Historically, ratiometric Ca^{2+}-binding dyes have been the gold standard in Ca^{2+} imaging experiments. Fura-2 has high Ca^{2+}-binding affinity, with a K_m of around 225 nM. The addition of an acetoxymethyl (AM) ester group improves membrane permeability. In our first studies of primary L and K cells, we used Fura-2AM to monitor nutrient-triggered Ca^{2+} changes. Fura-2AM loading of entero-endocrine cells in mixed primary cultures, however, proved difficult. Epithelial cells from the gut grow in partial monolayers, and isolated entero-endocrine cells are rarely found. Agents such as dimethyl sulfoxide (DMSO), eserine, and Pluronic F-127 improved loading, but may modify cell health.

The recent development of GECI has revolutionized real-time Ca^{2+} imaging in entero-endocrine cells. In transgenic models with L or K cell targeted GCaMP3, the Ca^{2+} indicator is endogenously expressed, and dye-loading problems are avoided. We use a GCaMP3 reporter mouse strain that can be crossed with various Cre mice to target GCaMP3 expression to a specific cell type. GCaMP indicators are chimeric proteins consisting of a circularly permuted enhanced green fluorescent protein (GFP) module fused with calmodulin and M13 domains. Upon Ca^{2+} binding, the calmodulin and M13 domains undergo a conformational shift that de-quenches the GFP fluorophore, resulting in an increase in GFP emission. This allows for a real-time readout of Ca^{2+} transients in single cells by monitoring the rise and fall of GFP emission. GCaMP3 has a K_m for Ca^{2+} binding of 660 nM.

To validate the use of GCaMP3, experiments were performed to monitor intracellular Ca^{2+} levels using Fura-2 and genetically encoded GCaMP3 in parallel (Fig. 2.3). Fura-2 and GCaMP3 signals were found

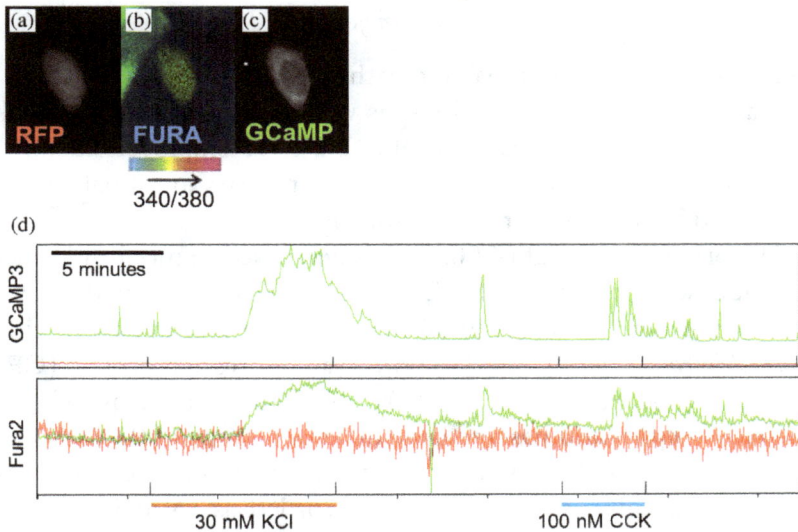

Figure 2.3.   Simultaneous imaging of intracellular Ca^{2+} levels as recorded by Fura-2 dye and genetically encoded GCaMP 3. Stomach cells isolated from mice expressing tdRFP and GCamP3 specifically in somatostatin-producing cells were plated on glass bottom dishes and imaged 24–48 h after plating. Cells were loaded with 5 μM Fura-2. D cells were identified by their red fluorescence (A) and were excited with 340/16 nm and 380/8 nm (B), and 488/8 nm (C). Cells were perfused with saline containing either 30 mM KCl or 100 nM CCK as indicated by the horizontal bars. Intracellular Ca^{2+} levels were represented by the 340/380 ratio, as measured by Fura-2, or intensity at 488 nm as measured by GCaMP 3 (D). The green lines indicate intracellular Ca^{2+} measurements from the selected cell; the red lines indicate background fluorescence.

to respond similarly to a range of stimuli, and the cell-specificity of GCaMP3 expression allowed for better signal-to-noise, as only the target cells display GCaMP3 fluorescence. Imaging of a single entero-endocrine cell is possible even within a clump of neighbouring cells, using the GCaMP3 method. Mass-loaded mixed cultures are problematic not just because the background noise is higher, but also because some recordings are ambiguous as there is no reliable way to distinguish whether the signal recorded from the area of interest arises from the target cell or from a neighbouring cell above or below the plane of focus. Together these characteristics make GCaMP3 imaging our preferred method for measuring Ca^{2+} transients in primary gastrointestinal cells.

2.4.2.2. *Förster resonance energy transfer (FRET probes)*

To explore G protein signalling pathways coupled to elevation of cytoplasmic cAMP concentrations, as well as cellular glucose uptake, FRET-based probes are useful (Table 2.2). We employed adenoviral vectors to introduce the FRET sensors into primary intestinal cultures, or standard transfection protocols for model cell lines.

The probe FLII$_{12}$Pglu-700$\mu\delta$6 has been used to monitor intracellular glucose levels in L cells. This sensor, first developed by Wolf Frommer, is derived from the glucose/galactose binding protein of *Escherichia coli* (Mg1B), fused to both cyan fluorescent protein (CFP), and YFP. *In vivo*, FLII$_{12}$Pglu-700$\mu\delta$6 exhibits a K_m for glucose of approximately 600 μM, and has a reliable detection range of 0.05–9.6 mM glucose, which is in the physiological range for intestinal cells. Increases in cytoplasmic glucose levels can be recorded as an increase in the YFP/CFP emission ratio.

For the analysis of G$_s$-coupled nutrient signalling pathways, we used the FRET probe, Epac2-camps. This probe is based on the cAMP binding domain of exchange protein directly activated by cAMP (Epac) isoform 2. The FRET signal between CFP and YFP in Epac2-camps decreases when cAMP is bound.

Table 2.2.   Fluorescent indicators used for monitoring intracellular signalling.

Indicator	Excitation λ/Emission λ	Messenger/nutrient measured
Fura-2AM	Ex: 340/380 nm Em: 525 nm	Intracellular Ca^{2+}
GCaMP3	Ex: 488 nm Em: 535 nm	Intracellular Ca^{2+}
FLII$_{12}$Pglu-700$\mu\delta$6	Ex: 435 nm Em: 470/535 nm	Cytoplasmic glucose, allows evaluation of glucose uptake mechanisms
Epac2-camps	Ex: 435 nm Em: 470/535 nm	Cytoplasmic cAMP, allows readout of G$_s$ pathway activity

2.4.3 *Primary Intestinal Epithelial Cell Culture*

A pivotal development in analysing incretin cells was the successful culture of adult intestinal epithelial cells. This is achieved through isolating intestinal crypts that spread into monolayers in culture. Fluo-rescently labelled entero-endocrine cells are visible for up to 10 days in primary colonic cultures and for 2–3 days in small intestinal cultures. This culturing technique is suitable for GLP-1 and GIP secretion assays, as well as single cell real-time imaging/electrophysiology analyses. Mixed primary intestinal cultures can be generated from adult mouse intestine as follows:

(1) Euthanise the mouse following a Schedule 1 method (UK Home Office) and confirm death.
(2) Open the mouse abdomen ventrally and remove the intestine from below the gastric pylorus to the rectum. Store the tissue in ice-cold Leibovitz-15 (L-15) medium for transport.
(3) Flush away the luminal contents using a Pasteur pipette with phosphate buffered saline (PBS) containing $MgCl_2$ and $CaCl_2$. Open the stretch of intestine longitudinally and wash the luminal side thoroughly.
(4) Using a fine pair of forceps, remove the muscle layer.
(5) Mince the tissue into 1 mm square pieces using a surgical blade.
(6) Collect the minced tissue into a 50 mL conical tube and rinse it three times using 15 mL PBS for each wash.
(7) Once the tissue has been minced, move into a biological safety cabinet for the remainder of the procedure.
(8) Rinse the tissue a further 3 times with 10 mL of sterile PBS.
(9) Filter sterilise a 0.375 mg/mL solution of Collagenase (type XI) from *clostridium histolyticum* solubilised in Dulbecco's modified Eagle's medium (DMEM) containing 25 mM glucose through a 0.22 μm filter and warm to 37°C.
(10) Add 10 mL of warmed, filtered collagenase to the tissue in a 50 mL tube. Invert the tube six times and begin the digestion.
(11) Incubate tissue at 37°C for 10 minutes for colonic cultures, or 5 min for small intestinal cultures, with forceful agitation every 5 min. Remove the collagenase-containing medium, taking care to avoid disturbing any tissue. This medium should be checked for digested crypts under a light microscope. If single crypts are present, the removed collagenase is centrifuged at 100 rcf for

3 minutes, the supernatant removed, and the pelleted tissue resuspended in 10 mL of sterile, filtered 25 mM glucose DMEM.

(12) These steps are repeated with the remaining undigested tissue a further three times. The last 2 digestions are carried out for 15 min for colon tissue, and 10 min for small intestinal tissue. Generally, only digestion steps 3 and 4 contain single crypts.

(13) Resuspended crypt pellets are centrifuged at 100 rcf for 5 min. The pelleted crypts are then resuspended in 4–6 mL of 25 mM glucose DMEM supplemented with 10% (v/v) FCS, 100 units/mL penicillin, 100 μg/mL streptomycin, and 2 mM glutamine. For imaging studies, 35 mm glass bottom culture dishes coated with a 1:100 dilution of Matrigel (VWR International) are seeded with 200 μL of the crypt resuspension. For secretion studies, 200 μL of the crypt resuspension is seeded onto 24-well plates coated with a 1:100 dilution of Matrigel.

(14) Cultures are incubated at 37°C, 5% CO_2 overnight.

2.4.4. GLP-1 and GIP Secretion Assays

To assess the role of a nutrient or signalling pathway in modulating incretin secretion, we perform static secretion experiments using intestinal epithelial cell cultures plated in 24-well plates. For these experiments, standard saline bath solution is required. The formulation is found in Table 2.3.

Table 2.3. Standard saline bath solution for hormone secretion experiments.

NaCl	KCl	NaHCO$_3$	NaH$_2$PO$_4$	CaCl$_2$	MgCl$_2$	HEPES	pH
138 mM	4.5 mM	4.2 mM	1.2 mM	2.6 mM	1.2 mM	10 mM	7.4

Hormone secretion assays can be conducted on primary cultures 16–24 h after plating as follows:

(1) Wash cultures thoroughly in PBS four times.

(2) Add 250 μL of test reagent prepared in standard saline containing 0.1% fatty-acid-free BSA and 1 mM glucose to the designated wells.

(3) Incubate cells for 2 h at 37°C.

(4) After the incubation, remove the bath solution into a clean 1.5 mL tube. Centrifuge these "supernatants" at 4°C for 5 min

at 200 rcf to remove cellular debris from the secretion sample. Transfer supernatants to a clean tube and freeze on dry ice.

(5) Lyse the remaining cells in buffer containing 50 mM Tris-HCl, 150 mM NaCl, 1% IGEPAL-CA 630, 0.5% deoxycholic acid, and one tablet of complete EDTA-free protease inhibitor cocktail (Roche, UK) for 30 min on ice.

(6) After mechanical disruption, collect the cell lysate and centrifuge at 4°C for 10 min at 200 rcf. Transfer supernatants to a clean tube and freeze on dry ice.

(7) Assess the hormone content in both the secretion sample and the cell extract fractions using an appropriate immuno-assay.

   (a) For GLP-1, we use the active GLP-1 [GLP-1_{7-36} amide and GLP-1_{7-37}] ELISA kit from Millipore or the total GLP-1 assay from MesoScale Discovery, Rockville, USA.

   (b) For GIP, we use a total GIP ELISA (Millipore).

(8) Hormone content in secretion samples should be expressed as a fraction of the total (secretion and cell extract) of that hormone measured in each well.

2.4.5. *Single-Cell Real-Time Imaging*

To perform calcium or FRET imaging analysis, intestinal cultures are plated on glass bottom dishes. Our imaging experiments are performed on an inverted fluorescent microscope attached to a charge coupled device (CCD) camera. Excitation and recording are controlled using Metafluor software (version 7.6.5.0; MDS Analytical Technologies). Cells are imaged with a plastic perfusion chamber placed in the bottom of the cell dish to reduce the chamber volume to approximately 250 μL.

2.4.6. *Calcium Imaging*

2.4.6.1. *Ca^{2+} monitoring with Fura-2*

Calcium imaging experiments using Fura-2AM (Invitrogen, UK) require cells to be loaded first. Loading is easier in cells that have been maintained in culture for more than 3 days.

(1) Primary intestinal cultures can be loaded with 5 μM Fura-2 AM in standard bath solution containing 300 μM serine, 0.01% pluronic, and 10 mM glucose for 30 min at 37°C. After penetrating the cells, the AM ester group is cleaved from Fura-2 AM by cellular esterases, allowing Fura-2 to bind intracellular calcium.

(2) Remove loading solution and incubate cells in standard saline solution containing 1 mM glucose at room temperature for 15 min–30 min, to facilitate hydrolysis of the AM ester from Fura-2, thus trapping the dye within the cells.

(3) Insert the perfusion chamber, carefully place cells on the microscope stage and insert inflow and outflow. Start perfusion with standard saline solution containing 1 mM glucose at a rate of ~1 mL/min.

(4) Using a 40× oil-immersion objective, visualise cells using either the Venus or tdRFP tag, as appropriate.

(5) Once a cell is located, monitor intracellular Ca^{2+} levels in real time:

(a) Excite cells at 340 nm and 380 nm (emission 510/80 nm), and record images every 2 seconds, e.g. using a 75 W xenon arc lamp and a monochromator.

(b) Background-subtract recordings and represent the images as the 340/380 nm ratio.

(c) Perfuse cells with desired test reagents made up in standard saline solution and record fluorescence changes.

2.4.6.2. *GCaMP 3 Ca^{2+} monitoring*

Primary cultures from mice expressing the genetically encoded Ca^{2+} indicator are imaged in the same way as Fura-2-loaded cells with the following amendments:

• Cells do not require loading, and are simply allowed to equilibrate to room temperature in standard saline solution with 1 mM glucose.

• Imaging is possible in cells cultured only for short periods to allow adherence to the dish.

• To measure intracellular Ca^{2+} levels, excite cells at 488/8 nm and collect the emission at 535 nm.

2.4.7. *FRET Imaging*

The methods for FRET imaging experiments carried out using the FLII$_{12}$Pglu-700$\mu\delta$6 FRET glucose sensor and the Epac2-camps cAMP probe are similar to those described for calcium imaging. The sensors are introduced by adenoviral or standard transfection methods. Primary intestinal cultures are imaged 48–72 h post adenoviral transduction, and model cell lines are imaged 48 h after Lipofectamine 2000-mediated transfection.

(1) Allow cells to equilibrate to room temperature in standard saline solution containing 1 mM glucose
(2) Insert perfusion chamber and carefully place cells on microscope stage, insert the inflow and outflow and begin perfusing at a rate of ~1 mL/min. Locate cells.
(3) Excite cells at excited at 435/10 nm, e.g. using a 75 W xenon arc lamp and a monochromator. CFP and YFP emissions are separated using a beam splitter (e.g. Cairn Optosplit II Image splitter).
(4) Acquire the emissions at 470 nm (CFP) and 535 nm (YFP). Express changes in FRET by taking the YFP/CFP emission ratio.

2.4.8. *Electrophysiology*

Patch clamp experiments are performed on primary intestinal cell cultures that are plated on plastic-bottom 35 mm dishes 3–10 days prior to recording or on model cell lines plated 1–3 days prior to recording. The formulations for standard whole cell and perforated patch pipette solutions are indicated in Table 2.4. Both solutions need to be adjusted to a pH of 7.2.

(1) Allow cells to equilibrate to room temperature in standard saline containing 1 mM glucose.
(2) Pull microelectrodes from borosilicate glass and coat the tip in melted beeswax.
(3) Fire-polish the electrodes using a microforge. Pipette resistances should be 2.5–3 MΩ.

Table 2.4.   Standard pipette solution for patch clamp experiments.

	K_2SO_4	KCl	NaCl	Sucrose	HEPES	$MgCl_2$	Amphotericin	$CaCl_2$	EGTA	ATP
Perforated Patch	76 mM	10 mM	10 mM	55 mM	10 mM	1 mM	200 μg/mL	N/A	N/A	N/A
Whole cell	N/A	107 mM	N/A	N/A	10 mM	1 mM	N/A	1 mM	10 mM	0.3 mM

(4) Place plastic perfusion chamber in cell dish, insert inflow and outflow, and begin perfusing cells at ~1 mL/min.
(5) Fill microelectrode with relevant pipette solution, and form gigaohm seal on cell.
(6) Record desired parameters using a patch clamp amplifier.

2.4.9. *Transcriptomic Analysis*

In order to perform gene expression analysis, both GLU-Venus and GIP-Venus mouse lines are used to isolate pure populations of L and K cells, respectively. To pass intestinal epithelial cells through the FACS sorter, they can be digested to single cells as follows:

(1) Process the desired segment of intestine to 1 mm pieces as described for primary intestinal epithelial cell cultures.
(2) Dissolve 1 mg/mL collagenase (type XI) in Hank's balanced salt solution (HBSS) without $CaCl_2$ or $MgCl_2$.
(3) Add 20 mL collagenase solution to tissue, and incubate at 37°C for 30 min with gentle shaking every 15 min.
(4) Remove the digestion media, being careful not to disturb the tissue pellet, and triturate 20–40 times using a 5 mL pipette. Filter this solution using a 70 μm filter into 2 clean 15 mL conical tubes.
(5) Spin the 15 mL tubes at 300 rcf for 10 min. Resuspend both pellets with 5 mL HBSS, and triturate a further 20–40 times
(6) Add 20 mL fresh collagenase solution to the remaining tissue pieces and shake vigorously.
(7) Incubate tissue at 37°C for 30 min, with vigorous shaking every 15 min. By the end of the second digestion all tissue should be digested.
(8) Filter the collagenase solution through a 70 μm filter into 2 clean 15 mL conical tubes
(9) Spin and resuspend as for digest 1.
(10) Filter all resuspensions through a 40 μm filter to combine.
(11) Spin one final time as above, and finally resuspend the pellet in 5 mL HBSS.
(12) FACS sort cells into desired RNA extraction buffer (Fig. 2.4).
(13) Extract RNA and proceed to either qPCR, microarray, or RNA-seq gene expression analysis.

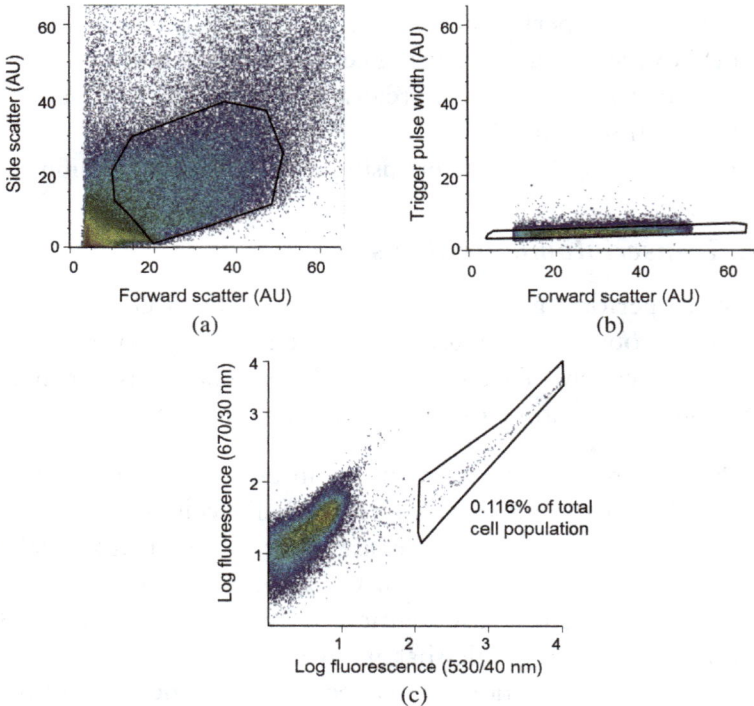

Figure 2.4. FACS purification of incretin cells. Intestinal epithelium from transgenic mice expressing the fluorescent protein, Venus, under the control of either the proglucagon or GIP promoter is digested to single cells. L or K cells are purified using flow cytometry. Cells are first gated based on their forward and side scatter to exclude debris and to isolate a subpopulation exhibiting the predicted size for incretin cells (A). This subpopulation is then gated based on trigger pulse width to isolate singlets to avoid contamination of the fluorescent population (B). Finally, L or K cells are purified from the singlet population based on their Venus fluorescence (C). These isolated incretin cell populations are sorted into buffer for RNA extraction and gene expression analysis.

2.5. Key Unmet Challenges

Through the use of adult intestinal epithelial cultures from transgenic mouse lines, we have begun to elucidate the cellular mechanisms underlying nutrient-mediated regulation of entero-endocrine cells. There is, however, a long way to go in our quest to understand how L and K cells are regulated *in vivo*, and how these mechanisms might be harnessed for the development of pharmaceutical solutions to combat the ever-growing burden of diabetes.

2.5.1. *Entero-Endocrine Cell Specificity*

Although traditionally seen as two separate entero-endocrine populations, the existence of a subset of cells expressing both GLP-1 and GIP has been well documented. The recent finding that entero-endocrine cells tagged through expression of fluorescent proteins under defined entero-endocrine hormone promoters show a more promiscuous hormonal profile than previously expected suggests some degree of plasticity in hormone expression within a closely related cell population. Given that entero-endocrine cells, like all intestinal epithelial cells, are derived from stem cells found in the crypts and have a short lifespan before they are shed from the villus tips, strategies to convert one cell type to another might prove therapeutically relevant. This cannot be simulated in the primary cultures described above, as no co-localisation of entero-endocrine cell-fluorescent tag and DNA-synthesis markers are observed, suggesting limited entero-endocrine cell differentiation under these conditions. The more recently described intestinal organoid cultures might, however, provide an *in vitro* model to address these questions.

2.5.2. *The Need for More Physiologically Relevant Models*

A limitation of our primary intestinal epithelial cultures is that the intrinsic polarity of entero-endocrine cells cannot be guaranteed. The disruption of cell architecture following the flattening of isolated intestinal crypts into monolayers, and prolonged periods in culture could result in the reorganisation of key cellular machinery, including glucose transporters and the cytoskeleton, which is integral to membrane trafficking and exocytosis. This displacement of cellular machinery could give rise to altered stimulus secretion activity.

In ideal circumstances, imaging experiments would be performed in freshly isolated tissue. Not only would this provide a more physiologically relevant environment to measure incretin cell activity, but it would also allow for the examination of the effect of cell location on intracellular signalling. For example, one would be able to investigate whether entero-endocrine cells at the tip of an intestinal villus are more potently regulated by nutrients than cells located deep in intestinal crypts. Though interactions between enterocytes and endocrine cells have already been proposed, efforts assessing whether a network of intercellular cross-talk exists in the intestinal villus would benefit from a recording system where cell connectivity and tissue architecture are intact. A system maintaining cellular and tissue polarity would also allow for real-time analysis of whether basolaterally applied nutrients and regulatory factors have implications for apically sensed nutrient signalling pathways.

A number of challenges are posed by the idea of developing an imaging system using intact segments of intestinal tissue. Not least is the difficulty of introducing nutrient and cell-signalling messenger probes into whole villi. The use of adenoviral vectors containing FRET probes to measure glucose or cAMP levels may be unrealistic given the amount of vector that would be needed to transduce whole segments of intestine. Additionally, commonly used GECIs are very dim when measured in intact tissue (unpublished observations). New mouse models and probes may be needed.

2.5.3. *The Need for Human Models*

Though experimental models based on murine tissue have been instrumental in furthering our understanding of incretin cell regulation, species differences are likely. In order for our current knowledge of nutrient sensing in L and K cells to be therapeutically relevant, experiments must be done to confirm the presence of putative signalling mechanisms in human incretin cells.

Recent advances in culturing techniques have allowed for the analysis of GLP-1 and peptide YY (PYY) secretion from human colon biopsies. These experiments confirmed that the elevation of cAMP is a key stimulus for incretin release, and also implicated polyunsaturated fatty acids and Gq-coupled pathways in human L cells.

This new ability for *in vitro* analysis of the human entero-endocrine system is encouraging. To enable transcriptomic analysis, however, further advances need to be made. Specifically, the identification of a reliable membrane-bound marker for L and K cells would make FACS-based analyses of human incretin cells possible. Antibodies against L- and K-cell-specific external antigens would facilitate the purification of live, unfixed cells for quantitative PCR, microarray, and RNA-sequencing. This would provide a means for assessing the value of current incretin cell models, as well as a database of potential targets for stimulating endogenous incretin release.

2.6. Conclusion

- The open-type morphology of L and K cells allows for direct nutrient sensing, and thus provides a critical link between the nutritional content of the intestinal lumen and the regulation of glucose homeostasis.
- Simple carbohydrates, products of lipid metabolism, amino acids and oligopeptides are potent secretagogues for incretin secretion.
- Entero-endocrine cells are electrically active, and fire action potentials when stimulated with glucose or amino acids.
- Key excitatory signalling mechanisms in L and K cells include electrogenic nutrient transport, and activation of G_s- or G_q-coupled GPCRs.
- Mechanisms underlying the direct regulation of incretin-releasing cells provide potential therapeutic targets for stimulating the endogenous incretin axis.
- Transgenic mouse lines expressing cell-specific fluorescent proteins and genetically encoded indicators provide versatile tools for transcriptomic and stimulus-secretion pathway analyses.

References

1. Gribble, F.M., Williams, L., Simpson, A.K. and Reimann F. (2003). A novel glucose-sensing mechanism contributing to glucagon-like peptide-1 secretion from the GLUTag cell line, *Diabetes*, **52**(5), 1147–1154.

2. Reimann, F. and Gribble, F.M. (2002). Glucose-sensing in glucagon-like peptide-1-secreting cells, *Diabetes*, **51**(9), 2757–2763.

3. Reimann, F., Habib, A.M., Tolhurst, G., Parker, H.E., Rogers, G.J. and Gribble, F.M. (2008). Glucose Sensing in L Cells: A Primary Cell Study, *Cell Metabolism*, **8**(6), 532–539.

4. Parker, H.E., Habib, A.M., Rogers, G.J., Gribble, F.M. and Reimann F. (2009). Nutrient-dependent secretion of glucose-dependent insulinotropic polypeptide from primary murine K cells, *Diabetologia*, **52**(2), 289–298.

5. Tolhurst, G., Heffron, H., Lam, Y.S., Parker, H.E., Habib, A.M., Diakogiannaki E., Cameron, J., Grosse, J., Reimann, F. and Gribble F.M. (2012). Short-chain fatty acids stimulate glucagon-like peptide-1 secretion via the G-protein-coupled receptor FFAR2, *Diabetes*, **61**(2), 364–371.

6. Simpson, A.K., Ward, P.S., Wong, K.Y., Collord, G.J., Habib, A.M., Reimann, F. and Gribble, F.M. (2007). Cyclic AMP triggers glucagon-like peptide-1 secretion from the GLUTag enteroendocrine cell line, *Diabetologia*, **50**(10), 2181–2189.

7. Parker, H.E., Wallis, K., le Roux, C.W., Wong, K.Y., Reimann, F. and Gribble, F.M. (2012). Molecular mechanisms underlying bile acid-stimulated glucagon-like peptide-1 secretion, *Br. J. Pharmacol.*, **165**(2), 414–423.

8. Diakogiannaki, E., Pais, R., Tolhurst, G., Parker, H.E., Horscroft, J., Rauscher, B. Zietek, T., Daniel, H., Gribble, F.M. and Reimann, F. (2013). Oligopeptides stimulate glucagon-like peptide-1 secretion in mice through proton-coupled uptake and the calcium-sensing receptor, *Diabetologia*, **56**(12), 2688–2696.

Chapter 3

Studying Incretin Action on the Pancreatic β Cell

D.J. Hodson and G.A. Rutter

Section of Cell Biology, Division of Diabetes, Endocrinology and Metabolism, Department of Medicine, Imperial College London

3.1. Introduction

In mammals, pancreatic β cells provide the main source of circulating insulin, the hormone primarily tasked with regulation of blood glucose levels. In healthy individuals, glucose is transported into β cells by membrane-spanning glucose transporters (i.e. GLUT2 in mice, GLUT2 and GLUT1 in humans), before glycolysis to pyruvate and synthesis of ATP in mitochondria by the tricarboxylate (TCA) cycle. The increase in the ratio of cytosolic free adenosine triphosphate/adenosine diphosphate (ATP/ADP) blocks ATP-sensitive K^+ channels (K_{ATP}), resulting in membrane depolarisation and opening of voltage-dependent Ca^{2+} channels (VDCC). The ensuing Ca^{2+} influx then drives exocytosis together with K_{ATP}-independent or amplifying signals (e.g. cAMP).[1]

It is generally acknowledged that the gut-derived incretins, glucose-dependent insulinotropic peptide (GIP) and glucagon-like peptide 1 (GLP-1), provide one of the most powerful amplifying inputs to insulin release.[2] As discussed in Section 3.2.3, incretins act chiefly via the latter "potentiating" pathways, which require elevated levels of blood glucose. It is this dependency on glucose which means that incretins have a far lower propensity to provoke hypoglycaemic episodes than other commonly used pharmacological agents to treat type 2 diabetes, (T2D) including sulphonylureas.

Whilst the basic cellular and molecular mechanisms underlying incretin action at the single β cell level are reasonably well established, less is known about how these are targeted by the diabetic milieu to impair insulin secretion. In addition, most studies to date have focussed their efforts on rodent islets, and it is becoming increasingly apparent that major species-differences exist in incretin-regulated β cell function. Indeed, loss of the incretin effect is an early characteristic of T2D in man (see Chapter 7) and studies of incretin action at the β cell level are therefore pertinent for the treatment of this disease state.

As such, the aims of this chapter are to describe the state of the art regarding:

1) the signalling pathways engaged by GLP-1 and GIP in β cells;
2) the influence of GLP-1 on the dialogue between individual β cells within intact islets;
3) species-specificity of the incretin effect;
4) T2D risk allele-incretin axis interactions; and
5) emergent technologies for the interrogation of incretin action.

Where applicable, step-by-step experimental protocols will be detailed, equipping the reader with the latest tools for the functional dissection of incretin-signalling in the pancreatic β cell.

3.2. Review of the Field

3.2.1. *Incretin Signalling in Single β Cells*

GLP-1 and GIP bind their cognate G-protein coupled receptors (GPCR) located on the β cell membrane to evoke a range of cell responses. The GLP-1 receptor (GLP-1R) is $G\alpha_s$ linked (i.e. engages small GTP-binding proteins of the αs family). Ligand binding consequently increases the activity of adenylate cyclase (ADCY), the enzyme that catalyses 3′-5′-cyclic adenosine monophosphate (cAMP) formation using ATP as a substrate. However, and in addition, GLP-1R activation also engages cAMP-independent pathways activating phosphatidyl inositol 3′-kinase (PI3-K) to alter transcriptional responses (see Figs. 3.1 and 3.2). The latter may involve an autocrine loop whereby the stimulated release of insulin (or possibly insulin-like growth factor-2 (IGF2)) leads to the activation of the cognate tyrosine kinase receptors for these ligands (i.e. insulin or insulin-like growth factor-1 (IGF1) receptors, respectively). Subsequent phosphorylation on tyrosine of adaptor proteins including insulin receptor susbtrate-2 (IRS2) or Shc can then lead to the recruitment of PI3K to the plasma membrane and the generation of phosphatidylinositol 3,4,5-trisphosphate (PIP3). This, in turn engages signalling pathways involving protein kinase B/Akt and mammalian target of rapamycin, mTORC, leading to nuclear events which ultimately enhance growth and survival.

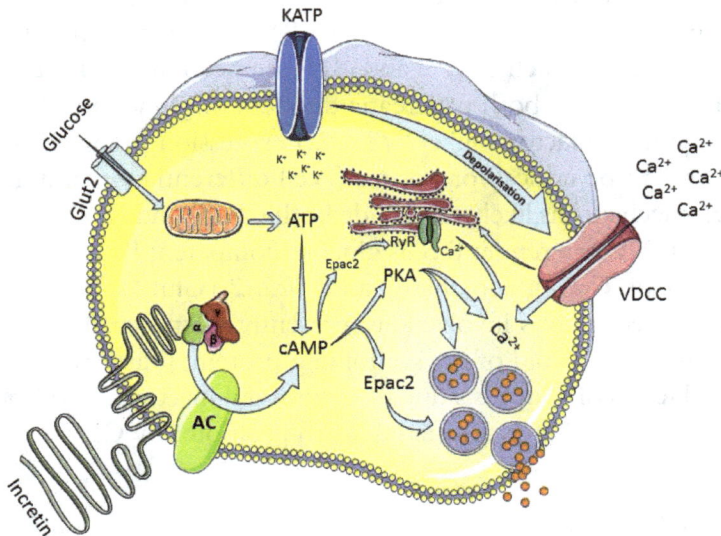

Figure 3.1.   Calcium fluxes engaged by incretins in beta cells. AC, adenylate cyclase; cAMP, 3′-5′-cyclic adenosine monophosphate; Epac2, exchange protein directly activated by cAMP 2; Glut2, glucose transporter 2; KATP, ATP-sensitive K⁺ channel; RyR, ryanodine receptor; VDCC, voltage-dependent calcium channel. Produced using Servier Medical Art with assistance from Mr. Ryan Mitchell.

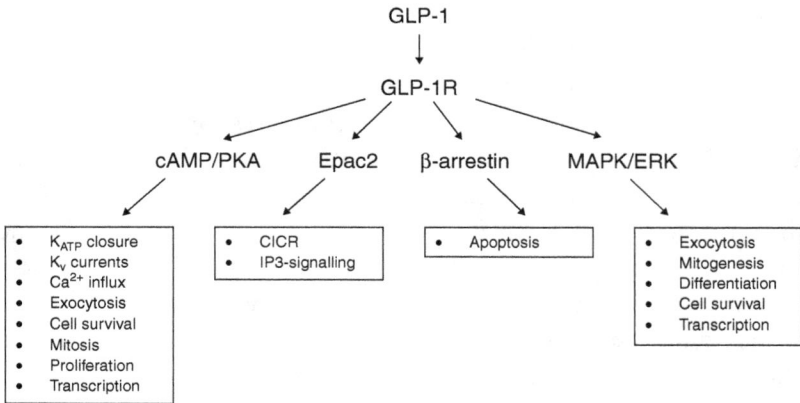

Figure 3.2.   Overview of GLP-1 signalling pathways in the β cell.

3.2.2. *Cell Survival and Apoptosis*

Increases in intracellular cAMP concentration result in the cAMP response element binding protein (CREB)-dependent transcription of key survival genes such as *Irs2* and *Akt* (see Section 3.2.1). Likewise, GLP-1 up-regulates both pancreatic duodenum homeobox-1 (*Pdx-1*) and transcription factor 7-like 2 *(Tcf7l2)* expression, transcription factors shown to be critical for normal β cell differentiation and growth, through mechanisms likely to include both CREB and RIS2 signalling. Finally, GLP-1 may render β cells glucose-competent by increasing the expression of *Gck* (glucokinase) and *Slc2a2* (Glut2), although the signalling mechanisms involved are presently unknown. Interestingly, islets from mice devoid of the scaffolding protein, β-arrestin 1, display increased levels of apoptosis due to diminished inactivation of the pro-apoptotic protein Bcl-2-associated death promoter by GLP-1.

3.2.3. *Ca²⁺ Influx*

In addition to the above, longer-term changes, incretins also act acutely on the β-cell (and note that, as described above, some of the tran-scriptomic effects depend on the more rapid responses that prompt the exocytosis of insulin and other growth factors). By prompting increases in intracellular cAMP, and consequently activating protein kinase A

(PKA), GLP-1 also inhibits K_{ATP} activity, potentiating the effects of glucose, which chiefly act on this channel by raising ATP/ADP ratios. This action of GLP-1 thus diminishes repolarising voltage-dependent K^+ currents, and increases calcium (Ca^{2+}) influx through VDCC. The net effects are increased sub-plasma membrane Ca^{2+} levels. These act on granule-bound Ca^{2+} sensors (notably small N-ethylmaleimide soluble factor-associated protein receptors or SNAREs, including synaptotagmin VII) to potentiate the exocytosis of insulin granules (Fig. 3.1).

3.2.4. *Intracellular Ca^{2+} Mobilisation*

GLP-1-induced elevations in cAMP also lead to the PKA-*independent* activation of exchange protein directly activated by cAMP (Epac). This guanine exchange factor (GEF) mobilises intracellular Ca^{2+} by sensitising the ryanodine receptor to Ca^{2+}-induced Ca^{2+} release (CICR) and, to a lesser extent, by evoking local increases in inositol trisphosphate (IP3) receptor signalling (Fig. 3.1). Importantly, GLP-1 is also thought to stimulate the synthesis of intracellular messengers capable of releasing Ca^{2+} from acidic intracellular organelles (lysosomes and secretory granules), creating microdomains of Ca^{2+} close to the plasma membrane. These may, in turn, lead to the opening of Ca^{2+}-activated non-selective cation channels (e.g. TRPM4 and TRPM5), contributing to the plasma membrane depolarisation that opens VDCCs (see Section 3.2.3).

3.2.5. *Exocytosis*

In addition to the above actions whereby GLP-1 increases intracellular Ca^{2+} levels, the incretin also improves the sensitivity of the exocytotic machinery in a Ca^{2+}- and K_{ATP}-independent manner (and animals lacking the SUR1 subunit respond normally to incretin). These effects are likely to involve GLP-1-induced changes in ATP, cAMP, PKA, and Epac2, the latter binding to granule-localised Rim2 and Piccolo. Lastly, mitogen-activated protein kinase (MAPK)/extracellular regulated kinase (ERK) signalling, which may be activated acutely though Ca^{2+}-dependent upstream kinases, has also been shown to increase insulin secretion. How MAPK interacts with the secretory machinery remains obscure, however.

3.2.6. *Cell Growth/Division*

GLP-1 is able to induce mitogenic/proliferative responses via phosphatidylinositol-4,5-bisphosphate 3-kinase- as described in Section 3.2.1, as well as through PKA-, protein kinase C (PKC)- and Ca^{2+}-dependent up-regulation of nuclear MAPK/ERK signalling. Nuclear factor of activated T-cells (NF-AT) signalling is also a likely further mechanism through which GLP-1-potentiated increases in intracellular Ca^{2+} act to stimulate β cell growth.

Similarly, GIP receptors (GIPR) are coupled to increased cAMP generation and GIP binding results in intracellular Ca^{2+} rises due to effects on VDCC activity, as well as activation of PI3-K, PKA, protein kinase B (PKB) and MAPK, as for GLP-1. In addition, GIP has also been shown to increase phospholipase activity, leading to hydrolysis of membrane phospholipid and liberation of arachidonic acid, a potent insulin secretagogue in its own right.

3.2.7. *Incretin-Modulated Energetics in Islets*

Whether and how incretins alter β cell metabolism to influence insulin secretion remains a source of contention. Early studies suggested that increases in cAMP, as prompted by incretins, were likely to have no effect on the oxidative metabolism of glucose. However, work over the past ten years has questioned this view. Thus, imaging with the ATP-sensitive recombinant probe luciferase has shown that GLP-1 increases mitochondrial ATP production in immortalised MIN6 β cells. On the other hand the GLP-1 mimetic, exendin-4 (Ex4), reportedly increases O_2 consumption in primary rodent islets without apparent effect on cellular ATP/ADP.

Further supporting a role for incretins in the control of β cell energy metabolism are the following observations:

- GLP-1 evokes large rises in intracellular free Ca^{2+} to potentiate insulin secretion.
- Ca^{2+} store refilling, active Ca^{2+} extrusion and exocytosis are energy-consuming processes that require net ATP production.

- Ca^{2+} entry into mitochondria stimulates the activity of citrate cycle dehydrogenases to up-regulate ATP synthesis.
- Excessive intramitochondrial Ca^{2+} concentration can disrupt ATP production by depolarising the inner mitochondrial membrane.
- GLP-1 activates hormone-sensitive lipases, which may increase ATP synthesis by promoting triglyceride breakdown and β-oxidation.

To resolve the question of a role for incretin in β cell metabolism, we have recently employed novel recombinant probes,[3] allowing the online measurement of ATP/ADP dynamics in the intact islet.[4] Using these approaches, GLP-1 triggers elevation and oscillations in ATP/ADP at both non-permissive (3 mM) and permissive (17 mM) glucose concentrations in rodent and human islets. This process is dependent upon GLP-1R binding and activated Ca^{2+}-influx through VDCC, and can be mimicked using forskolin to raise intracellular cAMP levels. Importantly, GLP-1-induced increases in ATP/ADP precede those of Ca^{2+}, as determined using multiparametric imaging of the nucleotide and ion. Therefore, GLP-1-stimulated insulin secretion is likely to require an augmented β cell metabolic set point. The previously reported differences in incretin action may stem from either the use of analogue (i.e. Ex4) versus native compound (i.e. GLP-1), or non-dynamic (i.e. luciferase assays in rodents) versus dynamic (i.e. Perceval) imaging measures. It is unlikely that such observations simply reflect compensation of ATP-consuming process (exocytosis, Ca^{2+} store refilling etc.), as Perceval measures the balance between ATP production and degradation. Figure 3.3 shows an updated model of incretin action on β cell energetics.

3.2.8. *Incretin-Regulated β Cell Connectivity*

There is little doubt that that the behaviour of individual, isolated β cells provides only a limited insight into the way these cells respond to stimulation within the intact islet. Importantly, the three-dimensional arrangement of β cells within islets appears to improve hormone secretion by encouraging the display of synchronous population activity,

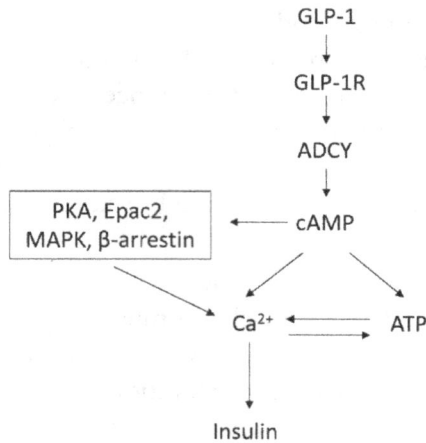

Figure 3.3.   Current view of GLP-1-regulated β cell metabolism.

as well as interactions with other islet non-β cells which may secrete β cell regulatory factors (glucagon etc.; though note that blood flow through the islet in the sense β-α-δ is thought to limit the action of the latter hormone on insulin release, at least in rodent islets). In contrast, β cells outside of their islet context are unable to properly coordinate their activities, resulting in inappropriately raised basal insulin secretion, as well as dampened responses to glucose. Thus, β–β cell intercommunication can be considered an essential element in the control of insulin release, and may represent an under-investigated target for T2D insults.

Using *in situ* imaging approaches allied to mathematical graph theory, we have recently shown that both GLP-1 and GIP recruit a highly coordinated subpopulation of β cells to boost glucose-stimulated insulin release.[5] This process, which we have termed "incretin-regulated connectivity", synchronises cell responses by promoting electrotonic (i.e. electrically modulated) gap junction (GJ)-mediated information transfer between β cell ensembles (Fig. 3.4).

Implying that incretin-regulated connectivity may be a target for pathological insults, and thus impair insulin secretion during insulin-resistance or T2D, islets from obese individuals fail to properly coordinate β cell activity in response to incretin. *In vitro* incubation with

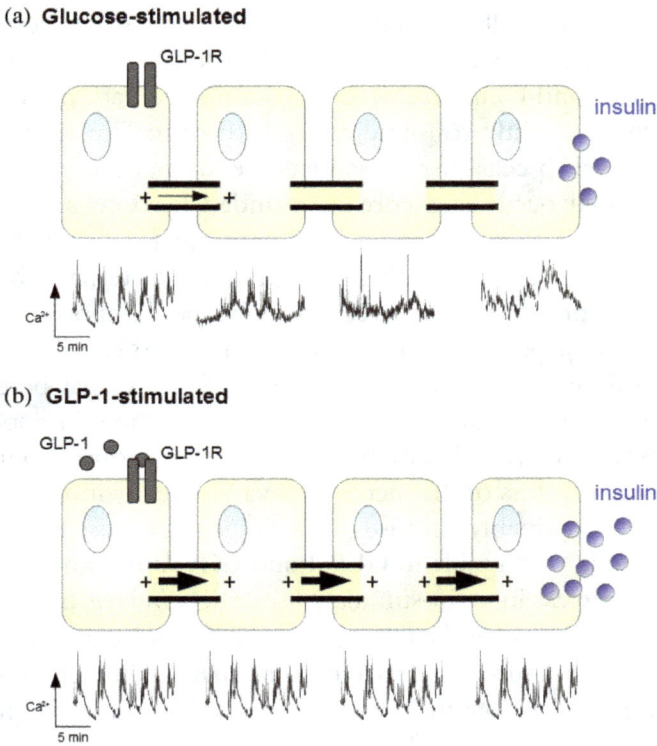

Figure 3.4. GLP-1-regulated β cell connectivity requires enhanced electrotonic cell–cell coupling.

palmitate mimics these findings, suggesting that the excess circulating free fatty acid (FFA) associated with obesity may impair normal glucose homeostasis in part by targeting normal β cell responses to incretin. Mechanistically, lipotoxicity reduces connexin 36 protein levels, the predominant GJ isoform that electrically links β cells, but does not affect either total or cell surface GLP-1R mRNA and protein expressions.

Remarkably, this phenomenon is not present in rodent islets, which usually present highly synchronous responses to glucose. On the other hand, this action of incretins on rodent islets can be unmasked by placing animals on a high fat diet (HFD; 60% kJ from fat) to disrupt GJ-mediated cell–cell communication. Such species-specificity of incretin action likely arises as a result of both dietary and structural influences.

Thus, rodents typically consume ~7% of calories as fat, compared to >20% for humans on a westernized diet. In addition, laboratory rodents are nocturnal and continuously graze during the dark phase, whereas humans intermittently consume meals at three to four sittings. At the structural level, β cells in rodent islets are arranged into a functional syncytium that occupies a core surrounded by α cells. By contrast, β cells in human islets are organised along laminar sheets, but appear to be intermingled with α and other cell types due to a tertiary-folding step during development. Thus, incretins may be more important in man as a signal to tailor peak insulin secretory demand to circulating glucose levels. In this respect, islets from the HFD-fed mouse may better model the human scenario due to disrupted daily rhythms in appetite and metabolism which reveal entrainment of β cell responses to incretin.

Importantly, loss of the incretin effect is an early indicator of T2D in humans, presumably because ~70% of insulin release following oral glucose load is attributable to GLP-1 and GIP. Although lipotoxicity is known to decrease incretin-stimulated secretion *in vivo*, this is generally considered to be secondary to glucotoxicity and decreased incretin release from the intestine. Our recent *in vitro* findings therefore suggest that excess circulating lipids may exacerbate glucose intolerance through primary effects on β cell responsiveness to incretin, supporting *in vivo* studies in which incretin action was impaired in obese individuals with normal glucose tolerance.

3.2.9. *Gene Variants and Incretin Action*

Genome-wide association studies (GWAS) have to date identified ~90 loci associated with T2D.[6] The gene locus with the largest effect on disease susceptibility is centred around *TCF7L2*, a transcription factor belonging to the canonical Wnt-signalling pathway. Notably, subjects harbouring the rs7903146 risk (T) allele present with markedly suppressed β cell responses to oral glucose tolerance tests (OGTT) (>50%), whilst secreting apparently normal levels of GIP and GLP-1. We have subsequently shown that silencing of *TCF7L2* expression in both rodent and human islets leads to decreased expression of GLP-1R and

GIP-R. Thus, genotype-incretin axis interactions likely play a major role in T2D risk in rs7903146 carriers. This notion is further reinforced by the finding that gene variants at the *GIPR* locus display a diminished incretin effect, as well as refractoriness to exogenously administered GIP, probably due to impaired *GIPR* transcript expression. It is worthwhile noting, however, that this SNP is weakly associated with T2D compared to *TCF7L2*, so defective GLP-1 function may play a relatively more important role in defining T2D risk. Interestingly, risk alleles in the ADCY5 locus, which encodes isoform V of the ADCY family, are not associated with impaired fasting glucose 2 h post oral glucose load. Moreover, we have shown that ADCY5 couples glucose but not GLP-1 to Ca^{2+} influx and insulin secretion via effects on cAMP generation and metabolism. Thus, the sugar and incretin engage distinct components of the cAMP pathway to potentiate insulin secretion. Such an arrangement may be advantageous due to parallel amplification of downstream effectors (i.e. PKA and Epac2), as well as increasing system robustness through multiple redundancy.

3.2.10. *Incretins and β Cell Growth/Apoptosis*

As well as their actions in insulin secretion, incretins also influence β cell survival.[7] Studies in rodents have demonstrated that both GIP and GLP-1 increase β cell proliferation, as well as protect against apoptosis. Such effects probably stem from a combination of signalling events, including the Irs2/PI3K/Akt, PKA/cAMP/CREB, ERK, β catenin-Wnt and β-arrestin pathways. Evidence for a similar role of the incretins in human β cell survival is much less convincing. Thus, whilst GLP-1 analogues restore glucose tolerance, this is unlikely to be due to any permanent effects on β cell mass, since symptoms reappear following treatment cessation. We note, however, that current means of estimating β cell mass in man provide only a very rough approximation and we await the development of imaging or other tools to quantitate this parameter more precisely.

The use of GLP-1 to increase human β cell proliferation *in vitro* has also been met with varying degrees of success; most workers have failed to see any evidence for enhanced proliferation.[7] Nonetheless, other studies have shown that GLP-1 prevents β cell glucolipotoxicity, and patients administered dipeptidyl peptidase-4 (DPP-IV) inhibitors to boost endogenous GLP-1 action display improved β cell mass, although some exocrine dysplasia was also noticed (see Chapter 8 for further discussion). However, the latter necessarily studied tissue from a small sample size.

3.2.11. *Using Recombinant Probes as a Readout of β Cell Status*

The advent of genetic-engineering has spurred the explosive development of recombinant probes or biosensors for the real-time measurement of β cell function. Key to this is the ability to clone non-native genes into viruses, allowing the expression of proteins that confer desirable properties upon mammalian tissue (e.g. fluorescence, light-sensitivity, energy-sensing etc.) Whilst biochemical assays remain the gold standard for assessing the effects of glucose and incretin upon signalling pathway activity, they are generally hindered by the requirement for a large number of cells, single time-point and single parameter measurements, and the challenges of targeting specific subcellular domains (e.g. the submembrane space versus cytoplasm versus mitochondrial matrix or endoplasmic reticulum lumen). To circumvent these drawbacks, bacterial, firefly, jellyfish and synthetic fusion proteins have been employed for the online monitoring of intracellular signals at the single cell and islet level.[3] Such probes are highly applicable to the dynamic measurement of responses to glucose and incretin, and pertinent members of this "genetically encoded signalling toolkit" are listed below.

- **Luciferase:** It can be expressed in cells as a recombinant protein but low light output means limited practical value without highly specialised detectors.
- **Perceval:** An ATP/ADP-sensing fusion protein consisting of Glnk1, a regulatory protein derived from the deep sea bacterium *Methanococcus jannaschii*, fused to a circularly permuted green fluorescent

protein (GFP). Binding of ATP closes the Glnk1 T-loop, leading to a conformational change and increased GFP fluorescence. Competition between ATP and ADP at the Glnk1 binding site allows the probe to act as a reporter of ATP/ADP ratio.

- **ATeams:** A FRET-based ATP sensor composed of cyan (CFP) and yellow (YFP) fluorescent proteins inserted either side of the bacterial F_0F_1-ATP synthase. ATP-binding leads to folding of the synthase ε-subunit, resulting in increased FRET and decreased CFP/YFP ratio.

- **Epac2-camps:** A FRET-based cAMP sensor consisting of a donor (CFP) and acceptor (YFP) fluorophore straddling the Epac2 cyclic nucleotide binding domain. Increases in cAMP lead to a decrease in FRET and an increase in the CFP/YFP ratio. Since CFP is pH-sensitive, and acidification can accompany depolarisation in excitable cells, newer Epac2-camps variants incorporate a relatively pH-insensitive cerulean/citrine FRET pair.

- **Flamindo:** An Epac1-citrine based cAMP sensor that displays a decrease in fluorescence intensity due to conformational changes induced by cAMP binding. It is well suited to super-resolution TIRF-imaging of cAMP compartmentalisation, as it displays a higher signal-to-noise ratio (SNR) versus FRET probes.

- **GCAMP:** A GFP-calmodulin-myosin light chain kinase (M13) fusion protein that acts as a genetically encoded Ca^{2+} indicator (GECI). Its primary advantages over chemical Ca^{2+} indicators (e.g. fura2 and fluo4) are the abilities to perform longitudinal imaging studies, and to target precisely to specified subcellular locales (see also Chapter 2).

- **VSFP:** Voltage-sensitive fluorescent proteins that use the conformational changes associated with voltage-sensitive phosphatase activity to alter FRET between donor and acceptor fluorophore pairs (e.g. mCitrine and mKate).

3.2.12. *Shining a Light on GLP-1-Regulated Connectivity Using Optogenes*

Optogenes are genetically engineered light-sensitive proteins that yield "remote control" over cell activity through alterations to membrane potential.[8] Although regarded principally as a neuromodulatory technique, optogenetics is equally applicable to electrically responsive endocrine cells, including β cells. In general, optogenes are light-responsive channels, pumps, or enzymes that allow the spatiotemporally precise manipulation of electrical or biochemical signalling events. To date, microbial opsins represent the most used class of optogenes and allow cell excitation or silencing by virtue of cation (Na^{2+} and H^+) or anion (Cl^-) influx (see Table 3.1). Opsin-adrenergic receptor chimeras also exist and allow the up-regulation of second messengers such as IP3 (β2-adrenergic) and cAMP (α1-adrenergic), although these are yet to be tested in β cells.

Two methods can be used to dictate expression of optogenes in pancreatic islets. The first uses the Cre-lox transgenic system to drive α- or β-cell-specific optogene expression. The second uses viral approaches and takes advantage of the fact that adenovirus is tropic for β over α cells. In both cases, optogene-expressing cells can easily be identified, since the ChR and NpHR constructs contain a fluo-tag with excitation-emission wavelengths orthogonal to those used for cell excitation and silencing. Opsin activation can be achieved using a conventional epifluorescence microscope and objective. However, it is recommended that fibre optic-coupled lasers or light-emitting diodes (LEDs) are employed to achieve the relatively high powers

Table 3.1.   Optogenes applicable for the manipulation of β cell activity.

Optogene	Format	Action	Ex λ (nm)	Tag
Channel rhodopsin (ChR)	Na^+ ion channel (light active)	Excitation	475	mCherry
Halorhodopsin (NpHR)*	Cl^- pump	Inhibition	585	EYFP
Archaerhodopsins (Arch-T)	Proton (H^+) pump	Excitation	550	EYFP
SwiChR	Na^+ channel (dark active)-	Inhibition	475	EYFP
iClC2	Cl^- ion channel	Inhibition	475	EYFP

*NpHR requires higher laser powers for activation than ChR.

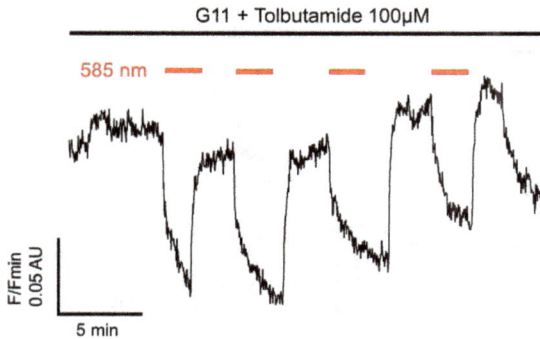

Figure 3.5. Reversible silencing of β cell Ca^{2+}-spiking activity using eNpHR3.0 (G11; glucose 11 mM). D.J.H and G.A.R. unpublished.

required for proper cell excitation/silencing, especially when targeting small regions at low magnification. An example of optical silencing of β cell Ca^{2+} spiking activity is shown in Fig. 3.5

We have recently begun to dissect functionally the islet wiring patterns which underlie β cell population responses to glucose and incretin. In particular, we have been able to show that some β cells contribute to glucose and GLP-1-evoked islet dynamics more than others (so-called "pacemaker" cells or "hub"). This "division of labour" is particularly interesting, since it challenges the traditional view that β cells represent a functional syncytium where all cells respond identically to a given stimulus. Indeed, such heterogeneity in response to input may reflect mechanisms to ensure robustness in the face of perturbation (e.g. diabetes) by maintaining a functional reserve. Alternatively, should insults repeatedly target this functional reserve, the consequences for tissue function would be catastrophic. Optogenetics holds promise for the precise interrogation of such wiring patterns. Indeed, ChR and NpHR can be used to yield pinpoint control over individual cells, allowing a role for glucose- and GLP-1-regulated pacemakers to be functionally explored, both under physiological and diabetogenic conditions (e.g. during obesity).

In Section 3.3, we provide protocols for the key imaging technologies used in our laboratories to study incretin-regulated β cell function.

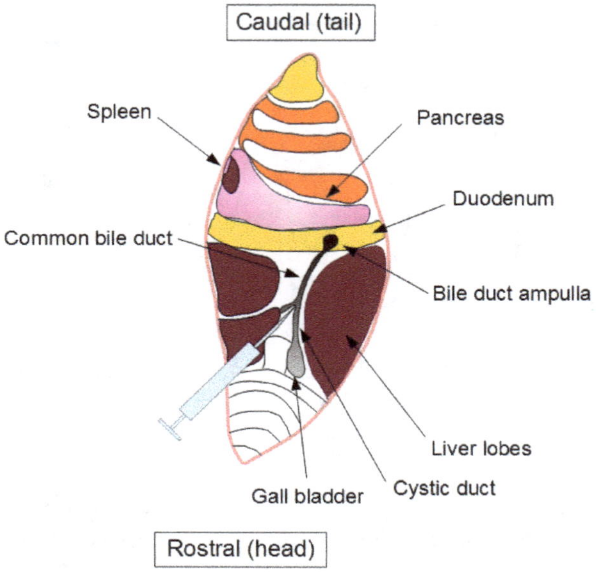

Figure 3.6. Landmarks and injection site for collagenase inflation of the pancreas in rodents.

3.3. Key Experimental Approaches

3.3.1. *Mouse Islet Isolation*

1. Euthanise the animal (CD1 or C57BL6 mice) using a designated UK Home Office Schedule 1 method and confirm death.
2. Perform an abdominal laparotomy under a dissecting microscope and clamp the bile duct ampulla where it enters the duodenum using mosquito forceps (Fig. 3.6).
3. With a 30 g needle, slowly inject 3–5 mL of collagenase solution (1 mg/mL in RPMI (Roswell Park Memorial Institute)) into the bile duct to inflate the pancreas (**n.b. if the pancreas doesn't inflate then withdraw the needle and advance more ventrally until solution traverses the bile duct lumen**).
4. Dissect out the pancreas and place into 3–5 mL of collagenase solution on ice pending digestion (**n.b. use a 50 mL "Falcon" tube to increase surface area for digestion; take care not to penetrate the gut!**).

5. Activate collagenase by placing tubes at 37°C in a water bath and incubate for 10 min **(n.b. depending on collagenase brand, you may need to perform a time series initially)**.

6. Stop reaction by adding 15 mL ice-cold RPMI. Centrifuge at 1000 rpm for 1 min before pouring off the supernatant. Add 15 mL RPMI and shake the tubes 20 times to dissociate the islets.

7. Wash the pellet twice with 15 mL RPMI. Centrifuge 1000 rpm for 1 min and discard supernatant.

8. Proceed to gradient separation. Add 3 mL Histopaque 1119 (1.119 g/mL polysucrose solution) to the pellet, mix using a plastic Pasteur pipette and transfer to a 15 mL Falcon tube. To the first layer, gently add 3 mL Histopaque 1083 (1.083 g/mL) followed by 3 mL Histopaque 1077 (1.077 g/mL). Finally top up until 12 mL using RPMI. Check that a sharply defined line is present between each layer **(n.b. it is critical to avoid mixing of the gradient interfaces!)**.

9. Centrifuge the gradient for 10–20 min, at room temperature, at 2500 rpm using maximum acceleration and minimum deceleration settings.

10. Recover islets that are present as a halo at the interface between the 1077 and RPMI layer and transfer to a 15 mL Falcon tube. Add RPMI up until 12 mL and centrifuge 1500 rpm for 3 min. Discard supernatant and resuspend islets in complete growth medium (RPMI +10% foetal calf serum +1% penicillin/streptomycin) **(n.b. avoid taking too much of the gradient otherwise final islet recovery will be reduced!)**.

11. Handpick islets into a 15 cm petri dish containing 10–15 ml of complete medium and incubate overnight at 37°C/5% CO_2 before commencing experiments.

3.3.2. *Functional Multicellular Calcium Imaging (fMCI) in Intact Islets*

1. Prepare HEPES-bicarbonate buffer (Table 3.2), saturate with 95% O_2/5% CO_2 and adjust pH to 7.4 using 1M NaOH. **(n.b. continued gassing is important to maintain pH!)**.

Table 3.2.   HEPES-Bicarbonate buffer constituents.

NaCl (mM)	KCl (mM)	NaH_2PO_4 (mM)	$NaHCO_3$ (mM)	HEPES (mM)	Glucose (mM)	$CaCl_2$ (mM)	$MgCl_2$ (mM)
120	4.8	1.25	24	5	3	2.5	1.2

2. Incubate islets for 30 mins with either 10 μM fluo2-AM (TEFLabs) or 10 μM fluo4-AM (Invitrogen) diluted with a mixture of 0.01% w/v DMSO and 0.001% w/v pluronic acid (20% stock solution in DMSO) **(n.b. incubate with fluo2/4 for 45 min max to avoid buffering of intracellular Ca2$^+$).**

3. Using a 200 μL pipette, carefully place islet(s) into a glass-bottomed imaging chamber containing buffer at 34–36°C. Incubate islets for a further 15 min to allow cytoplasmic esterases to cleave fluo2/4 into its active form **(n.b. do not add BSA to buffer otherwise the islet(s) will not adhere to the chamber!).**

4. Focus on the islet(s) using a 10× or 20× objective and deliver excitation at 470–495 nm. For best sensitivity and SNR, emitted signals should be recorded at 500–550 nm using an EM-CCD or CMOS camera **(n.b. use the fine focus to avoid damaging the chamber bottom with the objective).**

5. Deliver treatments via the perfusion system whilst imaging **(n.b. use a bubble trap to avoid movement artefacts due to air in the system).**

6. The sampling rate should be twice the highest frequency which needs to be resolved for analysis purposes (e.g. 4 Hz acquisition will be required to detect events at 2 Hz). To reduce artefacts associated with phototoxicity, reduce laser power and increase EM-CCD gain (i.e. let the detector do the work).

7. To resolve rapid events over a large area, high-speed imaging techniques will be required (e.g. spinning disk, resonant confocal and multibeam; see Fig. 3.7 and Table 3.3).

8. Traces can be represented normalised using the function F/F_0 where F is fluorescence at a given time point and F_0 is the minimum recorded fluorescence.

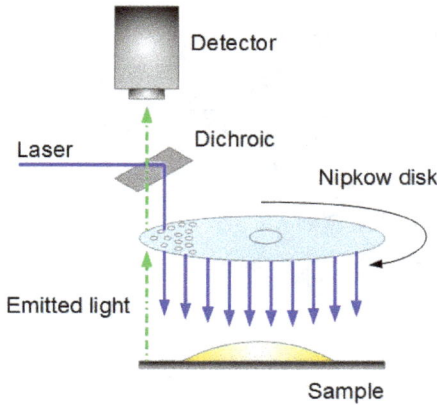

Figure 3.7.   The principles of Nipkow spinning-disk microscopy.

3.3.2.1. *Comparison of imaging approaches*

Table 3.3.   Comparison of different imaging modalities.

Imaging modality	Advantages	Disadvantages
Epifluorescence imaging	• Relatively cheap. • Scan area is only limited by detector sensitivity and size. • Speed is only limited by the exposure time required to adequately resolve a fluorophore. • Multiple wavelengths can be added simply by changing the excitation/emission filter. • Monochromator allows ratiometric imaging.	• Poor image resolution and penetration due to scattering and out-of-focus absorption. • Phototoxicity issues due to the large focal plane (axial and lateral). • No confocality so 3D images cannot be reconstructed without deconvolution algorithms.
Confocal laser scanning microscopy (CLSM)	• Pinhole blocks out-of-focus light which improves SNR and image resolution.	• High laser powers and/or pixel dwell times required to emit enough photons per pixel to resolve an image.

(Continued)

Table 3.3. (*Continued*)

Imaging modality	Advantages	Disadvantages
	• High resolution images due to use of photomultiplier tube (PMT) detectors. • Confocality allows 3D reconstructions.	• Use of PMTs limits quantum efficiency (QE), rendering Ca^{2+} events undetectable under dim light conditions. • Scan speed limited by pixel dwell time. • Depth penetration limited by out-of-focus absorption and scattering.
Nipkow spinning-disk confocal microscopy	• A rotating microlens splits the laser beam into beamlets which rapidly (ms) traverse a large area. • Large number of photons emitted during a single scan allows large areas to be rapidly imaged. • Low laser powers and pixel dwell time reduces phototoxicity.	• Use of an EM-CCD limits image resolution due to large pixel size. • Nipkow spinning-disk heads are expensive. • High transmission (up to 90%) loss requires powerful lasers. • Deterioration in quality at the image periphery
	• Use of an EM-CCD allows detection of event in dim-light conditions due to high QE. • Resolution of events into the kHz range; fluorophore intensity and detector sensitivity become limiting. • Lateral resolution identical to CLSM.	• Poorer axial resolution versus CLSM further limits imaging depth and resolution. • Back-reflected light and pinhole cross-talk can increase image SNR. • Unable to select a region of interest due to non-use of galvo-operated mirrors.
Two-photon confocal microscopy	• Similar to CLSM but uses a femtosecond-pulsed infrared laser to achieve the two-photon effect.	• Fluorophore excitation-emission spectra can become unpredictable in the infrared wavelengths range.

(*Continued*)

Table 3.3.   (*Continued*)

Imaging modality	Advantages	Disadvantages
	• The probability of a fluorophore simultaneously absorbing two-photons decreases inversely[2] with distance. Excitation outside of the focal plane is therefore unlikely. Decreases phototoxicity, increases SNR and increases depth penetration. • The infrared (>690 nm) wavelengths required for two-photon excitation are associated with less scattering versus those used for single photon imaging. Increases depth penetration and SNR. • Can be combined with second harmonic generation to study soft tissue structures (e.g. collagen).	• Femtosecond-pulsed lasers are large and expensive. • Mode-locked lasers introduce a delay when switching wavelength. • PMTs are required which limits QE. • Scan-speed similar to CLSM unless multiplexed systems are used. • Spherical aberration can degrade signal quality.

3.3.2.2.   *Comparison of Ca^{2+} indicators*

Table 3.4.   Ca^{2+} indicators commonly used for islet studies.

Indicator	Excitation/ emission	Notes
Fluo2/4	Exλ 488 Emλ 525	• Non-ratiometric • Good solubility in aqueous solution • Large dynamic range (~100-fold) • Good quantum yield

(*Continued*)

Table 3.4. (*Continued*)

Indicator	Excitation/ emission	Notes
Fura2	Exλ 340/380 Emλ 525	• Ratiometric • Leaks through Cl⁻ channels (non-leak version available) • UV excitation can be detrimental to cell function • UV excitation easily scattered
Fura Red	Exλ 440/470 Emλ 640-660	• Ratiometric • Poor quantum yield • Difficult to load into cells. • Can be combined with fluo2/4 to provide a ratiometric readout during confocal imaging (single wavelength spectrum: ex 488, emλ 640–660).
Indo-1	Exλ 340 Emλ 400/475	• Ratiometric • UV excitation can be detrimental to cell function • UV excitation easily scattered

Note: Fluo2 and fluo4 are well adapted for confocal techniques, since they can be excited by commonly-used laser lines, possess a K_d (~390 nM) compatible with β cell cytosolic Ca^{2+} concentrations, and display a large dynamic range. Fura2 may be preferred for epifluorescent microscopy, as it provides a ratiometric measure of intracellular Ca^{2+} rises, allows more accurate determination of Ca^{2+} concentrations, and is more compatible with other commonly-used fluorophores (e.g. EGFP and EYFP) (see Table 3.4).

3.3.3. *Dynamic ATP Imaging in Intact Islets*

1. Produce adenovirus-harbouring gene of interest (Fig. 3.8).[9]
2. Incubate islets for 48 h with adenovirus-harbouring Perceval cDNA at a multiplicity of infection (MOI) 10–100 (see Fig. 3.8 for construction). In our experience, this is sufficient to infect the first three islets layers, leading to widespread Perceval expression specifically in β cells. Non-β cells are poorly infected, probably reflecting low levels of viral receptors on these cells. However, titration should be performed for each batch of virus (**n.b. follow appropriate**

| 1. Excise gene of interest from plasmid | Restriction digest using *Eco*R1, extend using T4 DNA-polymerase and finally liberate using HindIII |

↓

| 2. Clone gene into pShuttlerCMV | Clone the Perceval-HindIII blunt insert into the EcoR1- and HindIII-digested pShuttleCMV |

↓

| 3. Transform HEK 293A cells | Split HEK 293A cells. Once 50% confluent, transform using a mix containing Lipofectamine 2000, DNA and GFP. Incubate for two days before splitting into 175 cm^2 flasks |

↓

| 4. Harvest virus | After 7–8 days, freeze-thaw three times to obtain particles without damaging the vector. Spin down at 4000 rpm and aliquot supernatant. |

↓

| 5. Amplify virus | Re-apply supernatant to fresh HEK 293A cells and harvest virus when cells detach. Repeat until the desired concentration is reacehd |

↓

| 6.Purify and concentrate virus | Sequential centrifugation in CsCl gradients before resuspending in a HEPES –MgCl-glycerol buffer. |

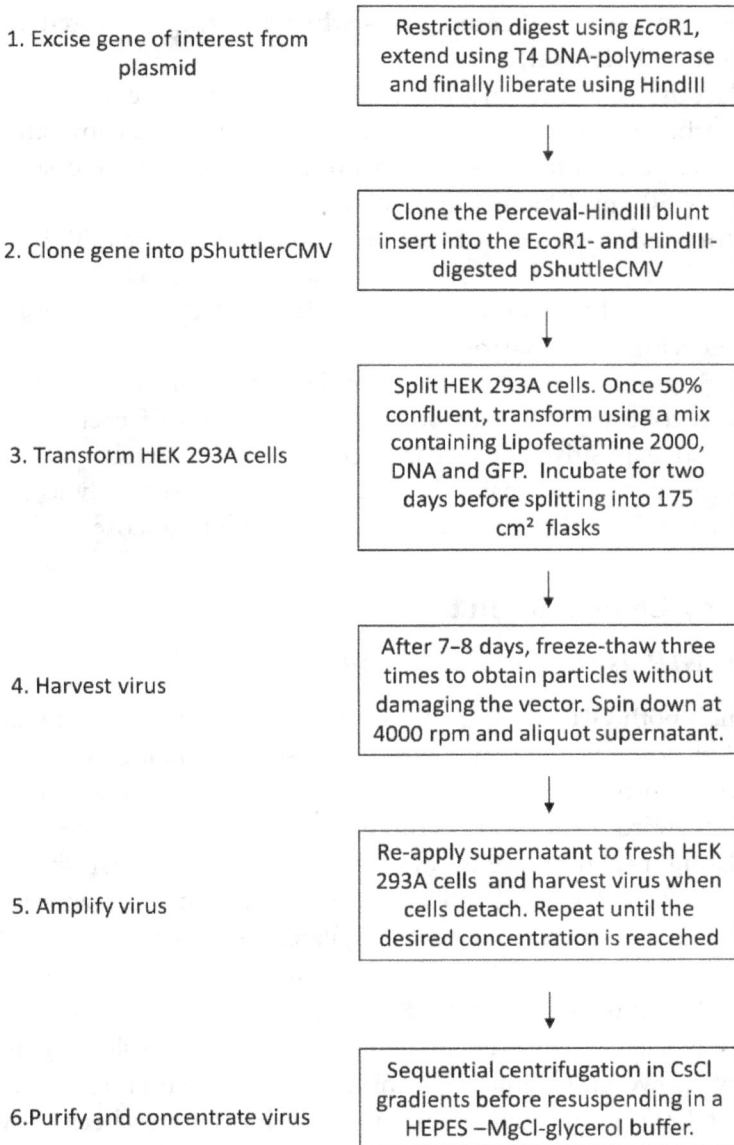

Figure 3.8.   Steps required to clone a gene into an adenoviral vector.[9]

local and national safety rules when working with genetically-modified viruses!).

3. Place islets in the imaging chamber and perifuse with HEPES-bicarbonate buffer containing the treatment under investigation. Deliver excitation at 470–495 nm and collect emitted signals at 500–550 nm. Changes in Perceval fluorescence intensity are oscillatory and slow (sec). Therefore, an acquisition rate of 0.2–0.5 Hz is sufficient to resolve ATP dynamics (**n.b. any effects of treatment on pH should be excluded, as GFP absorbs less light following protonation**).[3]

4. High glucose and carbonyl cyanide 4-(trifluoromethoxy)phenyl-hydrazone (FCCP) can be added at the end of each recording period as positive and negative controls, respectively.

5. Traces can be normalised using F/F_0, or alternatively as % F_{max}, where F_{max} is the maximum intensity at high glucose.

3.4. Key Challenges in the Field

3.4.1. *GIP as the Poor Relation*

Although both GIP and GLP-1 contribute to the insulin-raising actions of oral glucose, the incretin therapies licensed to date for use in humans fall firmly into the GLP-1 agonist category. The reason for this is straightforward: exogenously administered GIP is largely ineffective at stimulating insulin release during T2D. Whilst the mechanisms underlying diminished GIP action are poorly understood, it appears that *GIPR* mRNA expression is down-regulated by hyperglycaemia in both rodent and human β cells, most likely in a peroxisome proliferator-activated receptor gamma (PPAR-γ)-dependent manner. Of note, GIP responses can be restored in diabetic individuals following insulin therapy. However, whether GIP-mimetics could be useful for the treatment of T2D remains uncertain, since GIP infusion has been shown to decrease post-prandial glucose disposal due to stimulation of glucagon secretion. Therefore, further research is required to better understand:

1. how the diabetic milieu suppresses GIP effects;
2. the interactions between GIP and other endogenous insulinotropes to augment insulin secretion;

3. the influence of GIP upon α cell activity at various glucose concentrations; and

4. whether GIP signalling can be restored to counteract glucose intolerance during T2D.

3.4.2. *Intravital Imaging of Pancreatic β Cell Function*

The tissue microenvironment plays an important role in regulating insulin secretion *in vivo*. Indeed, β cells residing within islets of Langerhans are richly irrigated by a meshwork of capillaries which dynamically compensate the energy demands of actively secreting endocrine cells. In addition, the fenestrated vessels present in the islets may act as a rate-limiting factor in the uptake of secreted insulin into the circulation, as well as the delivery of tropic factors to the islet core. Thus, failure of the tissue microenvironment may play an underappreciated role in the β cell dysfunction associated with glucose intolerance and T2D. However, due to the location and friability of the pancreas, intravital imaging of β cells has historically been complicated by diaphragmatic excursions and the risk of pancreatitis. Recently, imaging studies have been described where islets are implanted into the immune-privileged anterior chamber of the eye, allowing stable and longitudinal imaging of islet function.[10] However, it is unknown whether the vascular-endocrine and exocrine–endocrine interactions present in the native pancreatic parenchyma are fully recapitulated in this setting. Therefore, demand exists for novel approaches that will allow the real-time monitoring of the islet environment *in vivo*, with the aim of understanding how this both influences and is influenced by incretin action.

3.4.3. *Incretin Signalling in Human Islets*

The majority of studies focused upon incretin signalling have employed either immortalised β cells or rodent tissue for reasons of practicality. However, the mechanisms underlying incretin-stimulated insulin are not conserved between species. Despite this, practically nothing is known about the signalling pathways engaged following GIP and GLP-1 binding in human tissue. For example, does GLP-1 predominantly operate using the classical Epac-camp pathway to direct intracellular

Ca^{2+} rises and exocytosis? Or are other pathways (e.g. involving MAPK and β-arrestin) relatively more important? Understandably, signalling studies in human tissue have so far been hindered by supply, as well as artefacts introduced by isolation method and transport distance. To this end, the recent availability of human β cell lines (e.g. EndoC-βH1), in combination with the GE-signalling toolkit described in the experimental approaches, may provide further clues about the identity of the molecular partners which link incretin to augmented insulin secretion.

3.4.4. *Incretin Action During Obesity*

The elevated circulating FFA concentrations associated with obesity drive glucose intolerance through suppression of insulin secretion, in addition to diminished insulin sensitivity. Whilst the negative effects of FFA on insulin and GIP receptor signalling are well documented, relatively little is known about whether links exist between obesity and impaired GLP-1 action. Suggesting that this may be the case are the observations that:

1. GLP-1-regulated human β cell connectivity is a target for lipotoxicity;
2. GLP-1 secretion is lower in individuals with high BMI; and
3. obese subjects with normal glucose tolerance still present with impaired GLP-1-stimulated insulin secretion, arguing against a role for glucotoxicity.

Therefore, it could be argued that T2D patients with BMI >30 who receive GLP-1 agonists (e.g. liraglutide and exenatide) demonstrate an initial normalisation of blood glucose levels due to the anorexigenic effects of such therapy. Given that obesity is the biggest risk factor for developing T2D, and incretin-mimetics are widely used as anti-hyperglycaemic agents, further studies are required to delineate the exact molecular and cellular mechanisms through which FFAs may reduce GLP-1 action.

3.4.5. *GLP-1R Distribution and Localisation*

Determining which pancreatic cell types express the GLP-1R has been challenging due to lack of an antiserum with sufficient sensitivity and specificity. It has now been shown that the majority of commercially-available antibodies, directed against various sequences of the GLP-1R protein sequence, are largely non-specific, since expression is still observed in tissue from GLP-1R$^{-/-}$ animals. Indeed, the reliable immunohistochemical detection of GPCRs is difficult, with antibodies directed against different epitopes frequently giving different results. Recently, a monoclonal antibody has been described which was produced by immunising GLP-1R$^{-/-}$ mice with purified human GLP-1R extracellular domain. This antibody has good specificity and confirms that expression of GLP-1R in human and primate tissue is largely co-localised with insulin, with some weak staining evident in acinar tissue. An alternative to immunostaining is the use of GLP-1 agonists tagged with a fluorophore. Whilst early examples lack the quantum yield required for detection without a secondary amplification step (i.e. an antibody against the fluotag), newer variants allow GLP-1R-expressing cells to be neatly highlighted. A particular advantage of such agonist approaches is that they allow β cells to be identified in live islets. Nevertheless, there is still demand for a panel of antibodies with specificity against the rodent GLP-1R, as well as inactive exendin-fluo analogues that do not interfere with β cell activity.

3.4.6. *Species Divergence in the Incretin Axis*

Marked heterogeneity exists in the structural and functional regulation of insulin secretion between species. As well as differences in the proportion and arrangement of α, β and other cells types, alterations to nervous and paracrine signalling are also apparent in human versus rodent islets. For example, insulin release from human islets is primed by a positive autocrine signal involving ATP liberated from insulin granules, and is under paracrine control by the neurotransmitter acetylcholine released from neighbouring α cells. By contrast, in rodent islets, ATP acts in a paracrine manner, and parasympathetic input is derived directly from nerve terminals. The impact that such signalling loops may have on GLP-1-stimulated insulin secretion remains unknown, but further investigation is warranted as they could provide the foundations for species-specific regulation of the incretin axis. A tantalising prospect would be that GLP-1, but not GIP, enrols a β cell → α cell signalling loop in human islets to exert its glucagonostatic actions. Likewise, the ability of GLP-1 to coax large-scale bouts of synchronous activity in a subpopulation of human β cells may partly stem from autocrine-mediated reinforcement of Ca^{2+}-spiking activity. In any case, the GLP-1R is predominantly expressed in insulin immunopositive cells, so any signalling interactions would need to emanate from GLP-1 action in the β cell. Finally, the relative importance of the direct effects of incretins on the β-cell, as described in this chapter, versus centrally mediated actions involving a central nervous system axis (see Chapter 5), also needs careful examination in suitable models.

3.5. Conclusions

- Incretin signalling in pancreatic β cells relies upon PKA, PKB, PKC, PLA_2, β-arrestin and MAPK pathways.
- Following activation of receptors on the β cell surface, incretins stimulate diverse effects in β cells including exocytosis, cell survival, cell proliferation, differentiation, and transcription.
- Incretin recruits a highly coordinated subnetwork of β cells to improve hormone release. Such incretin-regulated β cell connectivity is specific to human islets and is targeted by T2D insults.
- GLP-1 alters β cell metabolism, increasing ATP/ADP to support insulin secretion.
- Incretin-stimulated insulin secretion may be an important determinant of T2D risk in subjects harbouring risk alleles near gene loci, especially those for *TCF7L2* and *GIPR*.
- Recombinant probes allow the dynamic monitoring of the biochemical events underlying incretin action. Static assays may be unable to resolve changes to such parameters.
- Optogenetics provides a promising next-generation tool for understanding how glucose and incretin operate at the population level to produce a gain-of-function in insulin release.

References

1. Rutter, G.A., Pullen, T.J., Hodson, D.J. and Martinez-Sanchez, A. (2015). Beta cell identity, glucose snesing and the control of insulin secretion, *Biochem. J*, in press.
2. Campbell, J.E. and Drucker, D.J. (2013). Pharmacology, physiology, and mechanisms of incretin hormone action, *Cell Metabolism*, 17(6), 819–837.
3. Tarasov, A.I. and Rutter, G.A. (2014). Use of genetically encoded sensors to monitor cytosolic ATP/ADP ratios in living cells. *Meth. Enzymol.*, 542, 289–311.
4. Hodson, D.J., Tarasov, A.I., Gimeno Brias, S., Mitchell, R.K., Johnston, N.R., Haghollahi, S., Cane, M.C., Bugliani, M., Marchetti, P., Bosco, D., Johnson, P.R., Hughes, S.J. and Rutter, G.A. (2014). Incretin-modulated beta cell energetics in intact islets of Langerhans, *Mol. Endocrinol.*, 28(6), 860–871.
5. Hodson, D.J, Mitchell, R.K., Bellomo, E.A., Sun, G., Vinet, L., Meda, P. Li, D., Li, W.H., Bugliani, M., Marchetti, P., Bosco, D., Piemonti, L., Johnson, P., Hughes, S.J. and Rutter, G. A. (2013). Lipotoxicity disrupts incretin-regulated human beta cell connectivity, *J. Clin. Invest.*, 123(10), 4182–4194.
6. Rutter, G.A. (2014). Understanding genes identified by genome-wide association studies for Type 2 diabetes. *Diabet. Med.*, 31(12), 1480–1487.
7. Thorens, B. (2013). The required beta cell research for improving treatment of type 2 diabetes, *J. Intern. Med.*, 274(3), 203–214.
8. Zhang, F., Gradinaru, V., Adamantidis, A.R., Durand, R., Airan, R.D., de Lecea, L. and Deisseroth, K. (2010). Optogenetic interrogation of neural circuits: Technology for probing mammalian brain structures, *Nature protocols*, 5(3), 439–456.
9. Luo, J., Deng, Z.-L., Luo, X., Tang, N., Song, W.-X., Chen, J., Sharff, K.A., Luu, H.H., Haydon, R.C., Kinzler, K.W., Vogelstein, B. and He, T.C. (2007). A protocol for rapid generation of recombinant adenoviruses using the AdEasy system, *Nature Protocols*, 2(5), 1236–1247.
10. Speir, S., Nyqvist, D., Cabrerar, O., Yu, Y., Molano, R.D., Pileggi, A., Moede, T., Köhler, M., Wilbertz, J., Leibiger, B., Ricordi, C., Leibiger, I.B., Caicedo, A. and Berggren, P.O. (2008). Non-invasive *in vivo* omaging of pancreatic islet cell biology. *Nature Med.*, 14(5), 574–578.

Chapter 4

Action of Incretins on the Pancreatic α Cell: Control of Glucagon Secretion

L. McCulloch, M. Godazgar, P. Rorsman and R. Ramracheya

Oxford Centre for Diabetes, Endocrinology and Metabolism,
Radcliffe Department of Medicine, University of Oxford

4.1. Introduction

Type 2 diabetes (T2D) is often characterised as the inadequate β cell response to increased insulin resistance in peripheral tissues. However, there is strong evidence to suggest that glucagon secretion from pancreatic α cells is also dysregulated in subjects with this disorder. T2D should therefore be viewed as a bihormonal disease characterised by both hypoinsulinaemia and hyperglucagonaemia and the contribution of glucagon to the pathological disease state should not be overlooked.[1]

Glucagon is a hyperglycaemic hormone that, following secretion from the pancreatic α cell, is able to increase hepatic glucose output via suppression of glycolysis and stimulation of gluconeogenesis and glycogenolysis. In healthy subjects, glucagon secretion from α cells is stimulated by hypoglycaemia and suppressed during hyperglycaemia, thus working synergistically with insulin to regulate blood glucose levels within a narrow physiological range (4–6 mmol/L). In patients with T2D, however, perturbations in the regulation of glucagon secretion have been observed. For example, patients with T2D exhibit elevated plasma glucagon levels in the fasting state whilst demonstrating impaired suppression of glucagon secretion in response to glucose.[2] Importantly, glucagon dysregulation has been shown to contribute to the hyperglycaemic phenotype. Of interest, patients with T2D have demonstrated a delayed suppression of glucagon secretion in response to an oral glucose challenge, whilst suppression after an intravenous infusion mimicked that seen in healthy individuals.[2] This suggests that factors secreted via the oral ingestion of nutrients may be vital to the regulation of glucagon secretion.

Incretins ubiquitously enhance glucose-stimulated insulin secretion (GSIS) in pancreatic β-cells but can modulate differential effects on α cells. Thus, glucose-dependent insulinotropic peptide (GIP), released from K cells of the duodenum and proximal jejunum in response to the rate of nutrient absorption, *stimulates* glucagon secretion. Conversely, glucagon-like peptide 1 (GLP-1), released in a bi-phasic manner from L cells of the distal ileum (see Chapter 2), has a potent *inhibitory* effect on glucagon secretion. Consequently, analogues of GLP-1, rather than glucagon-enhancing GIP, have attracted therapeutic interest. To date they are the only available therapeutics which are able to both lower blood glucose levels by stimulating insulin secretion as well as suppress glucagon secretion in patients with type 1 and 2 diabetes.

Evidence from both *in vitro* and *in vivo* studies has demonstrated the efficacy with which GLP-1, and its analogues, can suppress glucagon secretion. Thus, GLP-1 infusion in healthy male subjects caused an inhibition of glucagon secretion at both low and high doses. In these subjects plasma glucose levels were lowered as a result of a 30% reduction in hepatic glucose production as opposed to glucose clearance, suggesting a direct role of GLP-1 on glucagon secretion *in vivo*. Similarly, additional *in vivo* studies have utilised the GLP-1 receptor (GLP-1R) antagonist exendin 9–39 (Ex9), as a means of blocking the actions of GLP-1. In healthy volunteers, administration of an oral glucose challenge reduced plasma glucagon levels as expected.

However, following a glucose challenge in subjects treated with the antagonist Ex9, glucagon suppression was lost and a modest increase in glucagon levels was noted.[2]

These findings clearly demonstrate that GLP-1 is able to modulate α cell function and glucagon secretion *in vivo*. However, these original studies have not addressed whether the glucagon-suppressing actions of GLP-1 are mediated by a direct action on the α cell, or via a paracrine mechanism. It is well established that GLP-1 stimulates insulin and somatostatin secretion from the pancreatic β and delta cells respectively. Both of these hormones can directly suppress glucagon secretion and therefore it has been postulated that GLP-1-mediated suppression of glucagon secretion may be caused via a paracrine interaction.

However, there is now compelling evidence suggesting that GLP-1-mediated glucagon suppression occurs via a direct (autocrine) effect on the pancreatic α cells and not as a result of a paracrine mechanism. In this chapter we will discuss the evidence for and against this theory, as well as highlight some of the experimental approaches which have been employed to date. In addition, we will focus on the technical challenges faced when elucidating the underlying mechanisms of GLP-1 action on α cells and discuss the questions that remain unanswered in this field.

4.2. Review of the Field

4.2.1. *Action of GIP on the α Cell*

Although both GLP-1 and GIP contribute approximately 80% of the insulin secretory response to oral glucose, the action of GLP-1 and GIP on glucagon secretion differs. Unlike GLP-1, which inhibits glucagon secretion, GIP exerts a stimulatory effect on glucagon release. Thus, GIP binds to GIP receptors (GIPRs) on α cells and stimulates the secretion of glucagon via increases in intracellular cAMP. Recent studies have reported local GIP production in mouse and human α cells, by means of immunohistochemistry and measurement of GIP secretion in response to various secretagogues. Although the functional role of local GIP production by islet α cells is unclear, one suggestion is that constitutive GIP secretion from α cells under stimulatory conditions, e.g. during fasting, can prime the β cells for improved subsequent GSIS.[3]

In T2D, the ability of GIP to enhance GSIS is lost, possibly due to chronic desensitisation or down-regulation of the GIPR.[3] This finding, coupled with the observation that GIP stimulates glucagon secretion, has rendered GIP therapeutically unattractive. Therefore the remainder of this chapter will focus on the other major incretin hormone, GLP-1, and its effects on glucagon secretion.

4.2.2. *GLP-1R Expression on Pancreatic* α *Cells*

As mentioned above, the observation that GLP-1 mediates an effect on glucagon secretion *in vivo* has led many groups to investigate the mechanism of its action. To this end, attention has naturally focussed on determining whether the classical GLP-1 receptor, GLP-1R, is expressed in α cells.

GLP-1R is a member of the glucagon receptor family of G-protein coupled receptors (GPCRs). The receptor was initially cloned from a rat pancreatic cDNA library in 1992 but has since been shown to be expressed in multiple human tissues including lung, heart, and the GI tract. Expression of GLP-1R in pancreatic α cells has proven more difficult to establish and multiple experimental approaches have been utilised to address this fundamental question.

Using radiographic density measurements obtained 2 hours post islet isolation, GLP-1 was found to bind to α and δ cells. However, binding was higher in insulin-producing cells, indicating higher levels of GLP-1R on β cells. Interestingly, when performing the same experiments 12 h or 24 h post-culture, a three-fold reduction in the signal was observed in all cell types, suggesting that islet culture can significantly alter the expression of the GLP-1R.[2]

GLP-1R expression has been demonstrated reproducibly in β cells at both the transcript and protein level. By contrast, GLP-1R expression in α cells has proved more difficult to establish conclusively. Using *in situ* hybridisation and double and triple immunofluorescence, GLP-1R has been found to be restricted to insulin-containing cells in rodent and human islets. To confirm the specificity of the methodology, tissue sections from GLP-1R knockout animals were stained, confirming total lack of GLP-1R expression in tissues known to be positive for the receptor.[2]

More recent approaches have utilised antibody-independent methods to determine the expression profile of the receptor in islets. A study in 2010 by De Marinis *et al.* used a transgenic mouse model expressing the Venus fluorescent protein under the proglucagon promoter and islets isolated from these animals were flow-sorted to obtain a pure preparation of α cells. Comparative mRNA expression analysis demonstrated that both α and β cells express GLP-1R, but levels in α cells were only 0.2% of those detected in β cells.[4] Considerable effort has also been invested in generating a more specific antibody against the GLP-1R. Recently, Pyke and others have reported the generation of a monoclonal antibody, which has been extensively tested in both primate and human tissues. Thus, when tested in normal monkey and human pancreas almost total co-localisation of GLP-1R and insulin was observed, although expression was also thought to be present in a very small subset of non-β cells.[5]

To date, the techniques employed to determine GLP-1R expression have mostly relied upon antibodies that have been neither sufficiently sensitive nor specific. Gene expression studies using quantitative real-time PCR (RT-PCR) have also raised concerns regarding the reliability of the data generated. Messenger RNA expression analyses are performed by generating amplicons far smaller than the entire full-length transcripts. It should be noted that cells are often able to produce multiple non-coding mRNAs from a single DNA sequence. These transcripts may be detected by the same primers that detect the full-length mRNA, thus providing no means of discerning between the coding and non-coding transcripts.

In summary, the conflicting findings in the literature regarding GLP-1R expression in α cells may arise as a result of several factors ranging from the use of freshly isolated versus cultured islets, the use of rodents in contrast to humans, experiments performed on single cells or fixed sections, or the use of non-specific antibodies. However, the current transgenic animal model results, coupled with data from a highly sensitive antibody analysis, suggest that GLP-1R is expressed at least in some α cells, but at levels considerably lower than those expressed in β cells.

4.2.3. GLP-1 Evoked Inhibition of Glucagon Secretion via Paracrine Mechanisms?

As discussed in Section 4.2.2, the initial controversy regarding GLP-1R expression in α cells, with some studies having failed to observe any expression at all, led to the suggestion that GLP-1 regulates glucagon secretion via paracrine interractions in the islet. As GLP-1R expression is abundant in β and δ cells, and given the islet architecture and potential cross-talk between different cell types, it is possible that insulin and/or somatostatin and their derivatives could influence the actions of GLP-1 on α cells. Interestingly, however, infusion of exogenous GLP-1 into patients with type 1 diabetes, who were unable to secrete detectable amounts of C-peptide (equivalent to endogenous insulin), resulted in significant reduction in glucagon secretion. The suppression in glucagon levels was comparable to that seen in T2D patients, who were able to also produce a 20-fold greater increase in plasma insulin and C-peptide, suggesting that the GLP-1 effect is independent of insulin secretion.[2] Likewise De Heer *et al.* have demonstrated inhibition of glucagon secretion by GLP-1 at a low glucose concentration, at which basal secretion of insulin was very low or undetectable.[4]

Having discounted a paracrine effect of insulin, De Heer *et al.* proposed that the inhibition of glucagon secretion may be exerted via somatostatin. Somatostatin receptors (SSTRs) are present on the α cell, predominantly in the form of subtype 2 (SSTR2). In a perfused rat pancreas, these authors investigated the importance of somatostatin on GLP-1-mediated glucagon suppression via two independent methods. Firstly, SSTR2 was blocked using a selective antagonist, PRL-2903, whilst in an additional set of experiments the effects of somatostatin were prevented by immunoneutralisation with a somatostatin antibody. In the presence of GLP-1, glucagon secretion was suppressed whilst addition of the SSTR2 antagonist alone enhanced glucagon secretion. However, co-application of the SSTR2 antagonist and GLP-1 was able to reverse the inhibitory effects on glucagon secretion. In fact, levels of secretion remained equivalent to those observed when treated with SSTR2 alone. In light of these findings De Heer and colleagues reported that GLP-1 mediated its effects on glucagon secretion via somatostatin. Interestingly, however, the authors were unable to completely replicate their findings via somato-statin immunoneutralisation. In the presence of a somatostatin anti-body, GLP-1 was still able to suppress glucagon secretion, although levels were attenuated compared to control experiments.[4]

4.2.4. *Direct Mechanism of GLP-1 Action*

Consistent with other studies, several pieces of evidence from our own group indicate that the inhibitory effect of GLP-1 on glucagon secretion may not exclusively result from a paracrine somatostatin-mediated mechanism. Firstly, in isolated mouse islets we have shown that in the absence of glucose, when insulin and somatostatin secre-tion does not occur, GLP-1 can still inhibit glucagon secretion by ~50% (Fig. 4.1(b)). Second, GLP-1 is able to retain its inhibitory properties in the presence of CYN154806, a somatostatin-receptor-2-specific antagonist targetting the somatostatin receptors in α cells. Third, GLP-1 inhibits glucagon secretion in dispersed mouse α cells whereby cell-to-cell communication is minimal or non-existent, thus ruling out any potential paracrine interaction.[4]

Therefore we have proposed that GLP-1 acts directly on the α cell to inhibit glucagon secretion. Key to this model is the low GLP-1 receptor density on the pancreatic α cells (Fig. 4.1(a)). We thus propose that GLP-1 binds to the low number of GLP-1 receptors and causes a proportional activation of Gs-coupled membrane receptors, which leads to a small increase in intracellular cAMP production. Subsequent activation of protein kinase A (PKA) leads to PKA-dependent phos-phorylation of P/Q-type Ca^{2+} channels,[6] inhibition of their activity, and reduced exocytosis of glucagon-containing secretory granules. This is in contrast to adrenaline, which activates 100- to 1000-fold more G_s-coupled membrane receptors and thereby produces a larger

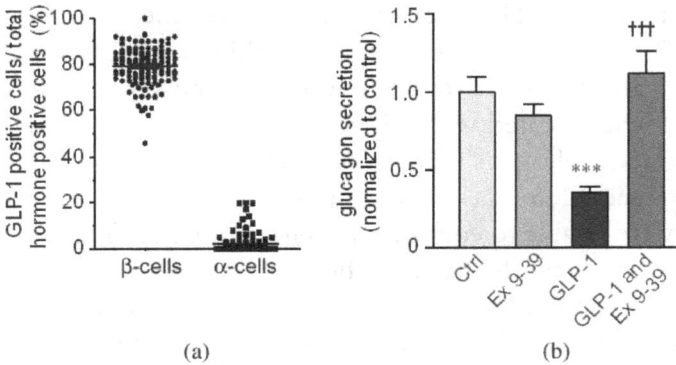

Figure 4.1. GLP-1R expression and GLP-1 activity in mouse islets. (a) Immunocytochemistry was performed for GLP-1R, glucagon and insulin in mouse islets. The number of β cells (insulin positive) and α cells (glucagon positive) which were also positive for GLP-1R are shown. (b) Glucagon secretion was determined at 1 mM glucose (Ctrl), in the presence of 100 nM GLP-1 and/or 1 μM exendin 9-39.[4]

increase in intracellular cAMP. Activation of the low-affinity cAMP sensor Epac2 binding, by the increase in intracellular cAMP concentration, leads to activation of L-type Ca^{2+} channels and increased Ca^{2+} influx, leading to enhanced secretion of glucagon. Interestingly, the differential effects of GLP-1 and adrenaline could be mimicked by low (nanomolar) and high (micromolar) concentrations of the adenylyl cyclase activator forskolin. Thus, low concentrations of forskolin inhibited glucagon secretion in contrast to high concentrations of the activator, which increased glucagon secretion.[4]

Although both glucose and GLP-1 mediate their inhibitory effects on glucagon secretion via the P/Q-type Ca^{2+} channel in mice, GLP-1 effects occur independently of the K_{ATP} channel. For example, use of the K_{ATP} channel activator, diazoxide, blocked the inhibitory actions of glucose but was not able to antagonise the effects of GLP-1. This suggests that glucose modulates P/Q-type Ca^{2+} channels by an indirect mechanism mediated by changes in the α cell membrane potential resulting from closure of the K_{ATP} channels, whilst GLP-1 inhibits glucagon secretion by a more direct effect on Ca^{2+} channel activity and exocytosis[4] (Fig. 4.2).

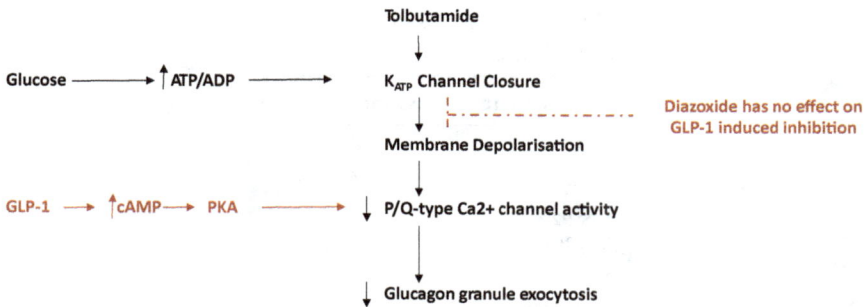

Figure 4.2. Glucose and GLP-1-mediated suppression of glucagon secretion in mouse islets. The effects of glucose on glucagon secretion are mediated via a K_{ATP}-dependent mechanism. These effects can be blocked by diazoxide, a K_{ATP} channel activator. In contrast, GLP-1 inhibits glucagon secretion by PKA-mediated inhibition of the P/Q-type calcium channel, bypassing the K_{ATP} channel.

The detailed cell physiological studies must now be validated to the same extent in human tissue. Preliminary work from our own group suggests that in isolated human islets, GLP-1 is able to directly mediate glucagon suppression. This effect is independent of the action of somatostatin, and can be blocked using the GLP-1R antagonist, exendin 9-39 (Ramracheya and Rorsman, unpublished).

4.3. Key Experimental Approaches

4.3.1. *Measurement of Insulin and Glucagon Secretion from Isolated Islets*

1. Prepare Krebs–Ringer buffer in advance as per Table 4.1. Adjust pH to 7.4 using 1M NaOH.
2. Supplement an aliquot of Krebs–Ringer buffer with glucose that would enable basal secretion of the major hormone of interest, for example 3 mM glucose for glucagon and 1 mM glucose for insulin.
3. Following isolation, pick 10–12 size-matched islets into 0.5 mL Eppendorf tubes containing 300 μL RPMI-1640 (in the absence of glucose). Wash the islets twice with RPMI.

Table 4.1. Krebs–Ringer buffer composition.

Constituent	Concentration
NaCl	140 mM
KCl	3.6 mM
$CaCl_2$	2.6 mM
$MgSO_4 \cdot 7H_2O$	0.5 mM
NaH_2PO_4	0.5 mM
$NaHCO_3$	2 mM
HEPES	5 mM
BSA	2 mg/mL

4. Pre-incubate the islets for 1 h in a wet chamber at 37°C in 300 μL Krebs–Ringer buffer. Following this time period, remove the pre-incubation buffer and discard.
5. Supplement Krebs–Ringer buffer with the test conditions at different glucose concentrations (i.e. 1 mM, 6 mM and 20 mM glucose) and add 300 μL to each tube.
6. Incubate the islets for a further hour in a wet chamber as in step 4.
7. Collect samples of supernatant (250 μL from each Eppendorf tube) for quantification of hormone secretion by radioimmunoassay (RIA).
8. Remove the remaining 50 μL supernatant *carefully* and discard. Supernatants are immediately frozen at –20°C to prevent degradation of the hormones, for later analysis by RIA. For insulin and glucagon RIA, follow protocols indicated by commercial kit providers.
9. Lyse islets in ice-cold acid ethanol solution (containing ethanol, H_2O and HCl in a ratio of 52:17:1) to release their hormone content.
10. Immediately store lysed pellets at –20°C.

4.3.2. *Identifying α Cells by Immunocytochemistry*

1. Rinse 0.17 mm coverslips three times in 95% ethanol before submerging in 0.1 mg/mL poly-L-lysine for 5 min. Place coated

coverslips at 37°C to dry before adding to wells of a 6-well plate. Cover the plates and sterilise before use.

2. Following islet isolation (described in Section 4.3.1), transfer cells to a 15 mL Falcon tube and remove excess media. Resuspend cells in 1 mL cell dissociation reagent and place in a water bath for 8.5 min. Add 10 mL RPMI (containing 10 mM glucose) to dilute the preparation before centrifuging at 130 × g for 5 min.

3. Remove excess media and resuspend the dissociated cell pellet in fresh RPMI media. Distribute 100 μL of cells directly into the centre of each coverslip. Incubate plates for 2 h at 37°C to allow cell adherence. Carefully add 2 mL RPMI to all wells and incubate overnight.

4. Aspirate culture media and fix the cells using 4% paraformaldehyde (for 20 min). Aspirate fixative and wash the cells twice with phosphate buffered saline (PBS).

5. To induce permeabalisation of the membrane, incubate the cells with 0.5% Triton-X (diluted in PBS) for 10 min. Perform 3 × 5-min washes with PBS. Prevent non-specific binding by blocking in PBS+BSA (bovine serum albumin) (1%) for 1 h (at room temperature).

6. Aspirate blocking buffer and add anti-glucagon primary antibody (diluted in blocking buffer). Incubate overnight at 4°C.

7. Aspirate off the primary antibody and wash the cells in PBS, 3 × 5-min washes (care must be taken to ensure cells do not dry out).

8. Incubate for 1 h with fluorophore-conjugated secondary antibody (must be performed in the dark). Aspirate the secondary antibody and perform 3 × 5-min washes in PBS.

9. Add mounting media to a microscope slide. Remove coverslips from six well plates and allow PBS to drip off. Place coverslips facedown onto the microscope slide and add clear nail polish around the coverslip to prevent the cells from drying out.

10. Examine slides under microscope using appropriate filters (dependent upon fluorophore conjugated to secondary antibody). Additional antibodies may also be included at steps 6 and 8 to allow identification of other cell types; i.e. comparisons may be performed between insulin positive and glucagon positive cells.

4.4. Introduction to Key Challenges

Elucidating the mechanism by which GLP-1 modulates glucagon secretion from the pancreatic α cell is fraught with several challenges, one of which is methodological. Currently there is an urgent need for a more robust detection system for many of the hormones and receptors involved in understanding the mechanisms of action of incretins.

In particular, although it has been more than 50 years since the glucagon RIA was developed, in general this field is still in its developmental stage and refinement of a robust and specific detection/assay system for glucagon, GLP-1 and GLP-1R is urgently needed. Current limitations on methodological approaches, namely sensitivity, specificity, reproducibility and reliability, may be contributing to different and often conflicting observations reported in the literature. To tackle this urgency, there is a current National Institutes of Health (NIH) call for the improvement of particular methods to help address such issues and a few such methods will be discussed here.

4.4.1. *Development of Specific Methods for GLP-1R Detection*

As mentioned in Section 4.2.2, many of the controversies surrounding GLP-1-mediated glucagon suppression to date have stemmed from inconclusive assessment of GLP-1R expression. Although variations may arise from different experimental approaches, there is also a certain amount of concern regarding reliability of commercially available detection methods. For example, pre-validated antisera detected non-specific bands when used on lysates from GLP-1R knockout mice whilst utilisation on lysates overexpressing GLP-1R failed to detect any immunoreactivity.[7] In a more recent study, three commercially available GLP-1R antibodies were used to determine GLP-1R expression in positive (normal mouse lung) and negative (mouse lung from GLP-1R knockout mice) control samples. The authors were not able to confirm the specificity or sensitivity of any of these antibodies.[7] Therefore, there is clearly a need to develop more extensively validated detection methods for the GLP-1R before we can fully understand its true expression profile. Although Pyke and colleagues have taken steps forward with the generation of their monoclonal antibody, this is likely to be an extremely challenging task due to the high levels of homology between GPCRs and their low cellular density.[5]

4.4.2. *Developing more Specific Antibodies for GLP-1 and Glucagon*

One of the key challenges facing researchers at present stems from the fact that both GLP-1 and glucagon are synthesised from the same precursor protein, proglucagon. This 158-amino-acid peptide is synthesised in both intestinal L cells and the pancreatic α cells. However, cell-specific cleavage events generate protein profiles unique to each cell type. For example, cleavage by prohormone convertase 2 (PC2) in α cells generates glucagon and major proglucagon fragment (MPGF) whilst predominant cleavage by PC1/3 in intestinal L cells generates GLP-1, GLP-2 and glicentin, which can itself be processed to glicentin-related pancreatic polypeptide (GRPP) and oxyntomodulin (Fig. 4.3).

Glucagon and GLP-1 are often detected in human serum or plasma. L cells and α cells are able to process the proglucagon peptide in tissue-specific manners before secretion. However, the generation of multiple proteins from one precursor peptide dictates the need for careful antibody selection to minimise cross-reactivity. Accurate quantification of plasma glucagon levels may be achieved using antibodies targeted to the N-terminus (amino acid 33) or to the C-terminus (amino acid 61). Unfortunately, N-terminus-directed anti-glucagon antibodies may also detect intestinally produced oxyntomodulin, whilst C-terminus-directed anti-glucagon antibodies can detect proglucagon 1–61. Similarly with GLP-1, antibodies directed to the N-terminus may bind to the MPGF secreted from the α cells whilst C-terminus antibodies will not be able to distinguish between the active (7–36) and inactive (9–36) forms of the metabolite. Therefore, antibodies targeted to one end of the peptide are unlikely to generate specific results when testing in plasma. One strategy would be to develop reliable and reproducible sandwich assays based on antibodies targeting both ends of the peptides.

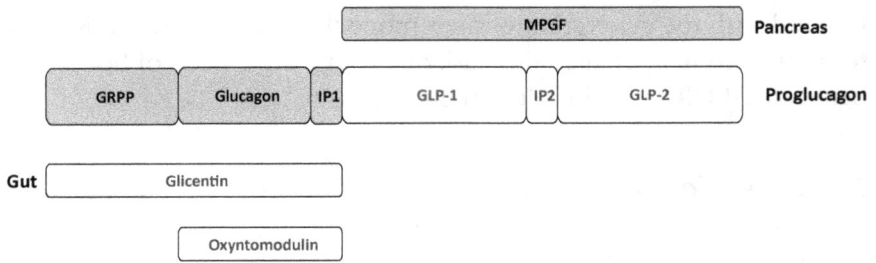

Figure 4.3. Structure of the proglucagon gene- and tissue-specific expression profiles. Within the pancreas, processing of the proglucagon gene by PC2 leads to the
generation of GRPP, glucagon, and the MPGF. Alternatively, processing within the
gut by prohormone convertases 1/3 leads to the generation of GLP-1, GLP-2 and,
glicentin, which can itself be cleaved to form oxyntomodulin.

4.4.3. *Rodent Islets versus Human Islets*

To date, much of the research into GLP-1-mediated glucagon suppression has been performed in rodent islets due to the scarcity of
human tissue. However, it is now well established that there are a
number of key differences between rodent and human islets. For
example, human islets contain fewer β cells (~55% of total cells) compared to rodent islets (70–80%), but in contrast possess a higher percentage of α cells (40% versus 20% for human versus rodent). Not
only do the two species contain varying proportions of endocrine cells
but their architecture has also been found to differ greatly. Thus,
rodent islets contain a core of β cells with an α cell mantle, whilst
human islets exhibit a trilaminar plate configuration. In humans,
β cells exist between two enriched α cell layers, but this structure is
able to fold into a configuration in which almost all endocrine cells are
in contact with the microvasculature, maintaining both homologous
β cell interactions and heterologous α–β cell connections. In addition,
a number of components of key signalling cascades have been shown
to differ between the two species. Thus, the threshold for glucose-
induced stimulation of insulin secretion is as low as ~3 mM in human
islets whereas glucose stimulation first becomes detectable at 6 mM in
mouse islets. There are also many differences in the complement of
voltage-gated ion channels and their density between human and

rodent islets (reviewed in Ref 8). These significant differences in the composition, structure, and function of islets indicate that they are regulated differently and it is important to consider these confounding factors when directly extrapolating data from one species to another. With a view to understanding the pathology in order to develop novel therapies for clinical diabetes it is therefore imperative that observations made in animal models are validated in human studies.

4.5. Introduction to Major Gaps in the Field

Despite global efforts to elucidate the role of GLP-1 on glucagon release, there remain several major gaps in this field.

4.5.1. *Gap #1: Is There a Second Receptor for GLP-1?*

As discussed in this chapter, a vast amount of work has been performed to elucidate the expression of the GLP-1R in pancreatic α cells. Despite evidence clearly demonstrating a direct action of GLP-1 on α cells, current highly sensitive techniques have shown receptor expression levels to be extremely low within these cells, totalling less than 1% of that observed in the pancreatic β cell and possibly concentrated on a few individual α cells. This phenomenon is also observed in other tissues throughout the body. For example, there is clear evidence of GLP-1-mediated effects on the liver, skeletal muscle, and adipose tissue and yet localisation of the GLP-1R in these tissues has remained inconclusive. This raises the question as to whether there may be an additional receptor via which GLP-1 is able to mediate its actions. GLP-1R belongs to the glucagon receptor family of GPCRs. These receptors share a similar conformation and are activated by ligands that are all derived from the same proglucagon precursor protein. It may therefore be tempting to speculate that a certain degree of cross-talk exists between these structurally similar ligands and receptors. In fact, one protein produced from the proglucagon precursor, oxyntomodulin, has already been shown to act as a partial agonist at the GLP-1R. Exploration of additional receptors for the GLP-1 ligand in future may provide additional insights into its mechanism of action on pancreatic α cells.

4.5.2. Gap #2: Evidence for a Local GLP-1 System in Pancreatic Islets?

One of the most striking aspects of GLP-1 is that only a small proportion of the active peptide secreted from the intestinal L cells is able to reach the pancreas, and yet GLP-1 has considerable functional activity on islets *in vivo*. This has led many groups to speculate as to whether there may be additional synthesis of GLP-1 locally within the islets, which could act in an autocrine manner to modulate islet function. A recent study by Marchetti and colleagues has used a combination of functional, molecular and immunohistochemical methods to address this question in human islets.[9] This group has convincingly shown that a small percentage (25%) of glucagon-positive cells co-stained with GLP-1 and that intact islets were able to secrete GLP-1 in response to a high glucose challenge. Islet GLP-1 content constituted a surprisingly large fraction of glucagon (25%), but it remains to be determined whether this represents biologically active GLP-1 or whether this signal is due to unspecific interaction with proglucagon components (it remains possible that the antigenic epitope is recognised by the GLP-1 antibody). Moreover, when conditioned media containing secreted GLP-1 was applied to an islet preparation in the presence of 11 mM glucose, GSIS was enhanced, an effect which could be blocked by Ex9. Importantly, GLP-1 did not localise to any insulin- or somatostatin-positive cells, which suggests that the local GLP-1 islet production is restricted to α cells.[9] However, although an up-regulation of PC1 (encoded by PSCK1) is likely to be central, other details regarding the molecular mechanisms underlying GLP-1 synthesis and secretion in α cells remain to be elucidated. In the future it will be important to determine how the proglucagon precursor peptide is processed to generate both GLP-1 and glucagon, and whether these hormones, with opposing biological functions, are packaged into distinct granules secreted in response to different stimuli. Moreover, it will also be pertinent to determine whether islets are able to synthesise and secrete dipeptidyl peptidase-4 (DPP-IV), the enzyme responsible for the cleavage of active GLP-1, and elucidate the role and activity of this enzyme in the islet milieu.

4.5.3. Gap #3: Is there a Role for GLP-1$_{9-36}$ in Islet Physiology?

The active form of GLP-1, GLP-1$_{7-36}$, has an exceptionally short half-life (see Chapter 1). Within minutes of entering the systemic circulation, GLP-1$_{7-36}$ is rapidly degraded to GLP-1$_{9-36}$ by the enzyme DPP-IV. Given that this breakdown product accounts for approximately 80% of systemic GLP-1, it has been argued whether this metabolite has any biological significance. Interestingly, however, in healthy human subjects, administration of GLP-1$_{9-36}$ was shown to have no effect on insulin response to glucose, glucose disappearance rate or glucose effectiveness in comparison to the active form of the incretin, which, in contrast, elevated each of these glucose homeostatic parameters.[10] These findings have been replicated by numerous groups and consequently GLP-1$_{9-36}$ has not merited any in-depth investigation as a potential regulator of glucose homeostasis and has since been deemed a "biologically inert" metabolite.

However, there is now emerging evidence from more recent studies suggesting that GLP-1$_{9-36}$ may be associated with a number of biological roles. Thus, intravenous administration of GLP-1$_{9-36}$ to anaesthetised pigs was shown to enhance glucose disposal by a mechanism independent of insulin secretion. Although the authors were unable to define the precise mechanism by which the effects were mediated, the study clearly demonstrated the effectiveness of GLP-1$_{9-36}$ to act as an anti-hyperglycaemic hormone.[10] Studies have also been performed to elucidate the effects of GLP-1$_{9-36}$ on peripheral tissues. During a euglycaemic clamp, administration of GLP-1$_{9-36}$ to obese subjects resulted in the need for glucose infusion as a result of a 50% inhibition of hepatic glucose production.[11] To further investigate the effects of GLP-1$_{9-36}$ on the liver, and to rule out a direct effect of insulin on gluconeogenesis, an additional study was performed in which isolated mouse hepatocytes were exposed to GLP-1$_{9-36}$ *ex vivo*. In the absence of insulin, the metabolite was still able to suppress gluconeogenesis in hepatocytes, confirming a biological role for the peptide.[11] In addition, recent studies have also identified a role for GLP-1$_{9-36}$ in cardiac function. GLP-1$_{9-36}$ is able to act as a vasodilatory agent, evoking cardioprotective effects in hearts isolated from

GLP-1R knockout mice and application of a DPP-IV inhibitor exhibited suppression of these cardioprotective effects.[11]

Therefore, in contrast to earlier reports, there is sufficient compelling evidence to redeem GLP-$1_{9\text{-}36}$ as physiologically relevant. Consistent with the earlier study, we have confirmed that GLP-$1_{9\text{-}36}$ does not affect glucose-induced insulin secretion but our preliminary data suggests that it is able to inhibit glucagon secretion in human islets with an efficacy as high as that of GLP-$1_{7\text{-}36}$ (Ramracheya *et al.*, unpublished). Although the molecular mechanisms by which this metabolite can suppress glucagon secretion remain to be established, fully understanding its role in glucagon secretion may lead to improved development of anti-diabetic agents. This, however, raises the argument that, if the breakdown product is essential for regulating glucagon levels, what will be the potential implications of DPP-IV inhibition therapy on its role?

4.6. Conclusion

GLP-1 is able to directly suppress the secretion of glucagon *in vivo*, making it a useful therapeutic treatment strategy. However, despite years of research, there remains a lack of consensus on the underlying mechanisms of GLP-1 action on α cells. Many of the conflicting reports in the literature are likely to have arisen due to the difficulties in assaying this highly homologous protein and the utilisation of non-specific antibodies. In the future, with the advent of more highly sensitive methodologies, it is hoped that these fundamental questions will be addressed. In addition, further characterisation of the local islet production of GLP-1 and biological significance of GLP-$1_{9\text{-}36}$ may lead to the development of novel treatment strategies for hyperglycaemia.

References

1. Unger, R.H. and Orci, L. (1975). The essential role of glucagon in the pathogenesis of diabetes mellitus, *Lancet*, **1**(7897), 14–16.
2. Holst, J.J., Christensen, M., Lund, A., de Heer, J., Svendsen, B., Kielgast, U. and Knop, F.K. (2011). Regulation of glucagon secretion by incretins, *Diabetes, Obesity & Metabolism*, **13**(Suppl. 1), 89–94.

3. Fujita, Y., Wideman, R.D., Asadi, A., Yang, G.K., Baker, R., Webber, T., Zhang, T., Wang, R., Ao, Z., Warnock, G.L., Kwok, Y.N. and Kieffer, T.J. (2010). Glucose-dependent insulinotropic polypeptide is expressed in pancreatic islet alpha-cells and promotes insulin secretion, *Gastroenterology*, **138**(5), 1966–1975.

4. De Marinis, Y.Z., Salehi, A., Ward, C.E., Zhang, Q., Abdulkader, F., Bengtsson, M., Braha, O., Braun, M., Ramracheya, R., Amisten, S., Habib, A.M., Moritoh, Y., Zhang, E., Reimann, F., Rosengren, A.H., Shibasaki, T., Gribble, F., Renström, E., Seino, S., Eliasson, L. and Rorsman, P. (2010). GLP-1 inhibits and adrenaline stimulates glucagon release by differential modulation of N- and L-type Ca2+ channel-dependent exocytosis, *Cell Metabolism*, **11**(6), 543–553.

5. Pyke, C., Heller, R.S., Kirk, R.K., Orskov, C., Reedtz-Runge, S., Kaastrup, P., Hvelplund, A., Bardram, L., Calatayud, D. and Knudsen, L.B. (2014). GLP-1 receptor localization in monkey and human tissue: Novel distribution revealed with extensively validated monoclonal antibody, *Endocrinology*, **155**(4), 1280–1290.

6. Rorsman, P., Ramracheya, R., Rorsman, N.J. and Zhang, Q. (2014). ATP-regulated potassium channels and voltage-gated calcium channels in pancreatic alpha and beta cells: Similar functions but reciprocal effects on secretion, *Diabetologia*, **57**(9), 1749–1761.

7. Drucker, D.J. (2013). Incretin action in the pancreas: Potential promise, possible perils, and pathological pitfalls, *Diabetes*, **62**(10), 3316–3323.

8. Rorsman, P. and Braun, M. (2013). Regulation of insulin secretion in human pancreatic islets, *Annual Review of Physiology*, **75**, 155–179.

9. Marchetti, P., Lupi, R., Bugliani, M., Kirkpatrick, C.L., Sebastiani, G., Grieco, F.A., Del Guerra, S., D'Aleo, V., Piro, S., Marselli, L., Boggi, U., Filipponi, F., Tinti, L., Salvini, L., Wollheim, C.B., Purrello, F. and Dotta, F. (2012). A local glucagon-like peptide 1 (GLP-1) system in human pancreatic islets, *Diabetologia*, **55**(12), 3262–3272.

10. Baggio, L.L. and Drucker, D.J. (2007). Biology of incretins: GLP-1 and GIP, *Gastroenterology*, **132**(6), 2131–2157.

11. Taing, M.W., Rose, F.J. and Whitehead, J.P. (2014). GLP-1(28-36)amide, the Glucagon-like peptide-1 metabolite: Friend, foe, or pharmacological folly?, *Drug Design, Development and Therapy*, **8**, 677–688.

Chapter 5

Role of Incretins in the Brain

J.E. Richards, S.C. Cork, M.K. Holt and S. Trapp

Centre for Cardiovascular and Metabolic Neuroscience,
Department of Neuroscience, Physiology & Pharmacology, UCL, London

5.1. Introduction

Glucagon-like peptide 1 (GLP-1) is best known for its effect as an incretin. It has a strong, glucose-dependent insulinotrophic effect, and thus limits post-prandial blood glucose elevation. This property has stimulated the use of stable GLP-1 analogues and inhibitors of GLP-1 degradation as safe anti-diabetic drugs (Chapter 8). During clinical studies, and since entering the market, pharmacological activation of GLP-1 signaling has, however, been found to have many additional effects including inhibition of glucagon secretion from pancreatic α cells (Chapter 4), positive effects on β cell mass (Chapter 3), cardiovascular protection and a sustained placebo-corrected weight loss. Whilst most of these effects are considered to be beneficial in patients with diabetes, undesired side effects include nausea and vomiting, especially at therapy initiation.

Interestingly, the incretins GLP-1 and glucagon-like peptide 2 (GLP-2) are not only produced in the gut (Chapter 2), but also within the brain and may have a function as neuropeptides, possibly independent from their incretin effects. Because the vast majority of research has been performed on GLP-1 rather than GLP-2, this chapter will discuss the effects linked to GLP-1 receptor (GLP-1R) activation in the brain, as well as the potential source of the GLP-1 acting on receptors in the central nervous system (CNS).

Most studies to date addressing the role of central GLP-1Rs in the regulation of blood glucose and appetite have employed intracerebroventricular (i.c.v.) injections of high concentrations of GLP-1 or a GLP-1R agonist. From these experiments it has emerged that not only the regulation of food intake by GLP-1 involves CNS targets, but also the control of blood glucose. However, at present the respective contribution of peripheral and central GLP-1 is unclear, as is the interaction of therapeutic GLP-1 analogues with the central GLP-1 system.

Should we be concerned about the potential effects of a neuropeptide GLP-1 on targets within the CNS? Would this be of any relevance for the use of GLP-1 analogues as anti-diabetic drugs? The answer is clearly yes. The CNS contains large numbers of GLP-1Rs, and these might be activated during GLP-1 therapy either directly, by GLP-1 analogues crossing the blood–brain barrier (BBB), or indirectly, by GLP-1 analogues acting in the periphery to generate afferent electrical signals. These signals in turn could activate GLP-1-producing neurons which project to cells expressing GLP-1Rs. Activation of central GLP-1Rs has pronounced effects on food intake, the control of blood glucose levels, blood pressure and heart rate. It also causes nausea, facilitates neuroprotection and can enhance learning and memory. These topics are addressed below.

Thus far, clinical observations have mirrored most of the findings from rodent studies: GLP-1 analogues act as an incretin, lower body weight and have a tendency to cause nausea or conditioned taste aversion. However, the hypertensive and tachycardic effects seen in rodents have not been reflected in human studies to date. This raises the question of how comparable the rodent and human GLP-1 systems are. The peptide itself is highly conserved between species, but information on the distribution of GLP-1-producing cells and GLP-1R-bearing cells in the human CNS is very sparse. However, two immunohistochemical studies, one on human and one on a non-human primate, suggest that the distribution of GLP-1-producing cells in the lower brainstem is very similar to that observed in rat and mouse, thus suggesting some validity of the rodents as a model system to study GLP-1 in the brain.[1,2]

As the vast majority of knowledge about central GLP-1 effects has been obtained from rodent studies, this chapter will review these. We present the key experimental approaches used to gain information about central GLP-1 effects and will finally highlight the major questions that are currently being addressed in the field. Whilst relying primarily on rodent studies throughout the chapter, there will also be references to the situation in man.

5.2. Review of the Field

5.2.1. *Role of Central GLP-1 in Regulating Food Intake*

The role of GLP-1 as a satiety signal has long been known, since activation of GLP-1Rs with peripheral administration of either the native ligand or the long-acting agonist exendin-4 (Ex4) significantly attenuates food intake in rats. Furthermore, removal of GLP-1R function by its antagonist exendin-9 (Ex9) has also been shown to increase feeding, adding weight to the argument that native GLP-1 is involved in the homeostatic control of feeding. What remains unclear is the exact role that central and peripheral GLP-1 plays in the regulation of food intake.

GLP-1 released from entero-endocrine cells into the circulation is rapidly degraded by the enzyme dipeptidyl peptidase-IV (DPP-IV). Therefore, although GLP-1 has been shown to cross the BBB, the rapid degradation, leading to a half-life of less than 2 minutes, might make any significant brain penetration unlikely, apart from at regions devoid of a BBB (i.e. circumventricular organs). It seems likely that CNS GLP-1Rs respond primarily to GLP-1 released within the brain and not from the gut. However caution should be taken when interpreting data obtained by peripheral administration of GLP-1 analogues, since these are not degraded by DPP-IV and thus might have a higher extent of brain penetration.

Within the CNS, GLP-1 is produced by a subset of neurons in the brainstem nucleus of the solitary tract (NTS), termed

preproglucagon (PPG) neurons. PPG, the precursor of GLP-1 and
glucagon, is expressed in these neurons because of the active glucagon promoter. Using a transgenic mouse model in which yellow
fluorescent protein (YFP) (Venus[TM]) is expressed under the control
of the glucagon promoter, it has been possible to map the projection
targets of these PPG neurons throughout the murine CNS
(Fig. 5.1).[3,4] A key finding from these studies is that brainstem PPG
neurons project widely to areas involved in homeostatic control of

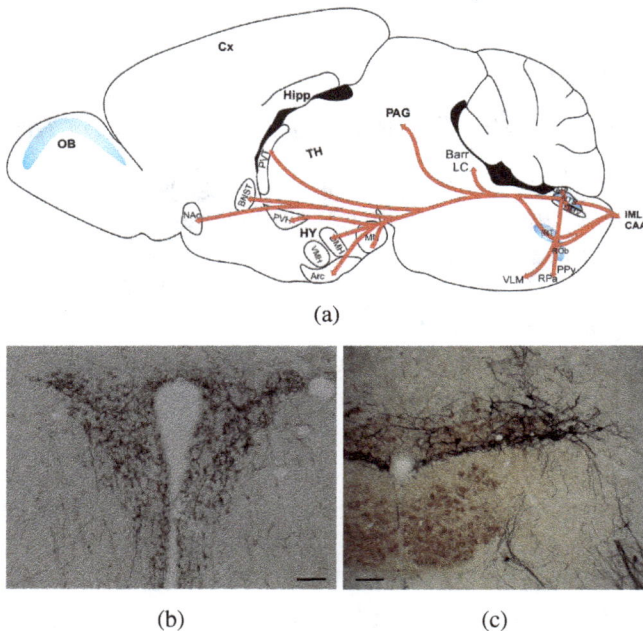

(a)

(b)   (c)

Figure 5.1.   GLP-1 is produced by PPG neurons located in the caudal NTS and
intermediate reticular nucleus (IRT), from which they project throughout the brain
with the notable exceptions of cerebellum, hippocampus (hipp) and cerebral cortex
(Cx). Such potential global control by GLP-1 may explain its suitability as a target
for drugs. (a) schematic drawing of a sagittal section through the mouse brain illus-
trating major projections of PPG neurons from the brainstem. Areas containing
PPG cell bodies are shown in blue. (b) microphotograph showing PPG axons
(black) in the PVN in hypothalamus from a mGLU-Venus mouse. (c) PPG neurons
(black) are located in the NTS adjacent to cholinergic (brown) dorsal vagal neurons
and hypoglossal neurons. Scale bars: 0.1 mm.

energy regulation, such as the hypothalamus, as well as areas associated with emotion and reward. This evidence supports their involvement not only in the autonomic control of energy homeostasis, but also in the emotional and psychological regulation of food intake. These strong projections are contrasted with the fact that the hippocampus, cerebellum and cortex do not receive PPG neuron innervation. Both globally and regionally there is a good correlation between the target areas for PPG axons seen in this mouse model and the distribution of GLP-1Rs examined by *in situ* hybridisation in rats. These transgenic animals have also allowed experimenters to directly record the electrical activity of identified PPG neurons *in vitro*. From these experiments, it has been shown that they are activated by exposure to the post-prandially released gut hormone cholecystokinin (CCK). That this activity was not the result of direct activation of postsynaptic CCK receptors on PPG neurons, but instead the result of increased inputs from glutamatergic neurons does not diminish the importance of the PPG neurons' role in satiety. Interestingly, the orexigenic peptide ghrelin failed to alter the electrical properties of PPG neurons, suggesting that satiation, and not hunger signals, are the driver of PPG neuronal activation. Furthermore, the adipocyte-derived hormone leptin increased the firing activity of PPG neurons. This discovery is important in solidifying the role of PPG neurons in the regulation of energy balance beyond short-term satiety signals, since leptin is a marker for the amount of fat stored by the body.

A further important observation from *in vitro* recordings of PPG neurons is that they receive monosynaptic inputs from vagal afferents entering via the solitary tract. Vagal afferent signals are known to send information regarding peripheral satiation to the brain as a result of both gastric distention following meal ingestion, and as a result of activation of receptors for peripheral satiation hormones, such as CCK and GLP-1. Whether vagal afferent signals to PPG neurons include those from gut-derived GLP-1, linking peripheral and central GLP-1 signals, is currently unclear and discussed further in Section 5.4. In any case, PPG neurons are in a prime position to respond to both immediate and long-term indicators of energy and feeding status.

Independently of whether the GLP-1 originates from PPG neurons or the gut, many studies have shown the importance of CNS GLP-1Rs in the regulation of food intake. Central injection of either GLP-1 or Ex4 has been shown to significantly attenuate food intake in rodents and results in the activation of neurons in hypothalamic nuclei involved in energy regulation.

One such area which shows increased activation following central injection of GLP-1 is the hypothalamic paraventricular nucleus (PVN). The PVN is an important site for control of the autonomic nervous system, and has particularly dense projections to sympathetic preganglionic neurons in the spinal cord. This allows the PVN to be in direct contact with the periphery and it is therefore an ideal centre for control of homeostasis. Known functions of the PVN include the control of energy and cardiovascular homeostasis. Anatomical studies have shown a dense innervation from PPG neurons as well as high levels of GLP-1R expression within the PVN. In rodents, activation of PVN GLP-1R by microinjection of GLP-1R agonists has been shown to result in a significant reduction in intake of normal chow and palatable high-calorie food for 24 hours. This is similar to the observations following activation of GLP-1R in the lateral hypothalamus, a site previously shown to respond to satiety signals. Interestingly, these results suggest that activation of these particular hypothalamic nuclei is sufficient to significantly affect feeding behaviour.

These results are in contrast to those observed for another hypothalamic nucleus, the arcuate nucleus (ARC). The ARC is regarded as perhaps the most important hypothalamic centre for regulation of energy balance, and its close anatomical relationship with the BBB-devoid median eminence places it in an ideal position to sample the peripheral energy availability. The ARC contains neurons, which synthesise either the orexigenic neuropeptide Y (NPY) and agouti-related peptide (AgRP) or the anorexigenic proopiomelanocortin (POMC) peptide, and studies have revealed a strong functional and anatomical connection between POMC neurons and GLP-1. Interestingly, however, activation of GLP-1R in the ARC has little or no effect on food intake, but does result in a significant inhibition of glucose production and increase in glucose uptake.

Perhaps one of the most interesting areas of research in the central GLP-1 system is the effects of GLP-1 on the mesolimbic reward system. Composed of nuclei including the ventral tegmental area (VTA), nucleus accumbens (NAc) and amygdala, the mesolimbic reward system is a network of nuclei involved in food and drug rewarding behaviours. Both the VTA and NAc contain high levels of PPG fibres originating from the brainstem and activation of neurons in these areas leads to a significant reduction in food intake, even in food-deprived animals. Surprisingly, freely fed animals given the choice between normal chow and high fat food showed a significant reduction in high-fat food intake following intra-VTA/NAc injections of Ex4. This was due to a reduction in meal size, with no change in normal chow consumption. Furthermore, activation of VTA or NAc GLP-1Rs reduces the motivation for palatable foods. These results make the mesolimbic GLP-1 system a tantalising therapeutic target for the control of overeating and obesity, since its modulation appears to preferentially control for high-fat palatable foods.

As well as a potential target for the control of food intake, modulation of the mesolimbic GLP-1 system has been shown to have potent effects on drug and alcohol intake. Peripheral administration of GLP-1 has been shown to decrease alcohol intake in rodents, an effect which was more potent when animals were separated into "high" and "low" baseline alcohol drinkers. GLP-1 activation had a more potent effect in "high" baseline alcohol consumers. Although the exact mechanism by which peripheral GLP-1 administration results in a reduction in alcohol intake remains controversial, studies have shown that injection of Ex4 into the VTA results in a significant reduction in alcohol consumption with no alteration in normal water consumption. In addition, rodents pre-treated with peripheral Ex4 were found to reduce their consumption of nicotine, cocaine and amphetamines compared to controls. This also correlated with a reduction in NAc dopamine levels. These results provide enticing evidence that therapeutic targeting of GLP-1R in the mesolimbic reward system may provide not only an effective treatment for obesity, but also for alcoholism and drug abuse.

5.2.2. *Role of Central GLP-1 in Thermoregulation*

In addition to its well-defined role in regulating the feeding state of animals, it is becoming increasingly evident that central GLP-1 has a role in regulating the metabolic activity of brown adipose tissue (BAT). The primary role of BAT is to provide heat through non-shivering thermoregulation. Both GLP-1 and Ex4 potently increase BAT temperature when injected i.c.v. This is accompanied by an increase in BAT sympathetic activity and genes associated with thermoregulation. Retrograde tracing studies have shown that BAT sympathetic innervation originates from hypothalamic centres, including the ventromedial hypothalamus and PVN, as well as the mesolimbic bed nucleus of the stria terminalis. Innervation was also found in the intermediolateral cell column of the spinal cord, an area known to contain large numbers of sympathetic preganglionic neurons. Importantly, all these areas have been shown to receive innervation from brainstem PPG neurons.

Interestingly, results from human studies suggest that increases in the metabolic activity of adipose tissue in response to GLP-1 treatment may be responsible, at least in part, for a decrease in fat mass and an increase in resting energy expenditure independent of physical activity levels.[5] These results suggest that GLP-1 may have the ability to alter basal energy levels through mechanisms other than regulating food intake. This is of particular therapeutic interest, since activation of BAT thermogenesis could be beneficial for the treatment of obesity in the absence of any lifestyle changes.

5.2.3. *Role of Central GLP-1 in Cardiovascular Regulation*

The therapeutic potential of GLP-1 analogues makes it paramount to understand their cardiovascular effects, and findings thus far look promising. GLP-1 has been shown to be cardioprotective and antihypertensive. In patients with type 2 diabetes (T2D), a decrease in blood pressure was observed following 48 hours of continuous GLP-1 infusion. However, in a randomised double-blind placebo control study, no significant difference in either heart rate or blood pressure was observed after 12 weeks of Ex4 (exenatide) treatment (for review see[6]). The antihypertensive effect has been linked to activation of GLP-1Rs located on cardiac myocytes. In contrast, a number of studies in rodents have demonstrated that both peripheral (i.v.) and central (i.c.v.) administration of GLP-1R agonists caused acute hypertension and tachycardia. Interestingly, prior blockade of central GLP-1R with the antagonist Ex9 prevented this. Furthermore, i.c.v. administration of a vasopressin antagonist prevented the rise in blood pressure, but not heart rate associated with i.c.v. GLP-1 infusion, while bilateral vagotomy also ablated the effect of central GLP-1 infusion. Similarly, it has been reported in a mouse model that GLP-1R activation reduces heart-rate variability via inhibition of parasympathetic outflow. Collectively, these results suggest that both sympathetic and parasympathetic arms of the autonomic nervous system may be responsible for the cardiovascular effects of central GLP-1. If the results from further clinical trials are found to match those observed in rodents, we would argue that GLP-1 actions in the CNS might be detrimental for diabetic and/or obese patients suffering from hypertension and/or heart disease.

5.2.4. *GLP-1 and Nausea*

One of the most significant limiting side effects of therapeutically administered GLP-1 analogues is nausea. This symptom is seen in both human and rodent studies and limits the effectiveness of and tolerance to these drugs. The cause of GLP-1-induced nausea is not fully understood; anatomical studies of PPG neuron projections could provide some clues. Brainstem PPG neurons send descending projections and make putative synapses with serotonergic neurons in the brainstem. These serotonergic neurons in turn send ascending projections back to the dorsal vagal complex (DVC), a collection of nuclei including the NTS and dorsal motor nucleus of the vagus (DMNX) that has been implicated in the physiology of nausea and vomiting. Since 5-hydroxytryptamine (5-HT) 3 subtype receptor ($5\text{-}HT_3$) activation within the NTS has been implicated in nausea, it is possible that GLP-1-based therapies activate GLP-1R on serotonergic neurons, which in turn release 5-HT to activate 5-HT$_3$ receptors within the DVC. This is, however, speculative and further research needs to be undertaken to understand the physiology behind GLP-1-induced nausea in order to increase the efficacy of GLP-1-based therapeutics.

5.2.5. *Glucose-Dependent Insulinotropic Polypeptide (GIP)*

Unlike GLP-1, significantly less work has been undertaken examining the role of glucose-dependent insulinotropic polypeptide (GIP) as a neuropeptide. Within the CNS, GIP has been implicated in roles that include neuromodulation, neuroprotection and neurogenesis, as well as modulation of food intake, body weight, and core body temperature. GIP immunoreactivity and mRNA have been detected in many brain areas including the hippocampus, thalamus, PVN, DMH (dorsomedial hypothalamic nucleus), amygdala and cortex, and autoradiography has identified GIP binding sites throughout the brain.

Although little work has been undertaken on the role of GIP as a central regulator of energy homeostasis, the existing work is conflicting in nature. Chronic administration of GIP into the lateral ventricles of rats resulted in a significant reduction in weight gain compared with control-injected rats. Conversely, vaccine-induced antibodies directed against GIP, which reduce its endogenous availability, when administered *in vivo* also resulted in a reduced weight gain compared to controls as well as a decrease in hippocampal and cortical glucose utilisation. Consequently, more studies are needed to ascertain whether central GIP contributes to the regulation of energy homeostasis and if so, to what extent.

5.3. Key Experimental Approaches

Characterising a peptidergic system in the brain presents several challenges. How does one identify cells producing the peptide or recognise cells expressing the peptide receptors? Which methods should be used to study these cell populations functionally? And finally, how can one manipulate the system *in vivo*? Most of these challenges can now be addressed thanks to advances in genetics and molecular biology.

5.3.1. *Determining the Distribution of GLP-1 and GLP-1 Receptors in the CNS*

GLP-1 is produced by posttranslational processing of the product from the glucagon gene. Transgenic mice have been generated by using regions upstream from the coding sequence of the glucagon gene to drive expression of fluorescent marker proteins. Interestingly, the first of these strains showed expression of the fluorescent marker only in pancreatic α cells that produce glucagon and not in the gut or the brain where GLP-1 is expressed. Only in the second strain (mGLU-Venus), generated by Reimann and colleagues, where the transgene incorporated a much larger fragment of the upstream sequence of the glucagon gene, was YFP (Venus™)-fluorescence observed in the appropriate cells in gut and brain.[7] This has allowed detailed characterisation of the PPG neurons in mice as described in Section 5.2.1.

Another mouse model from the same laboratory employs a knock-in of the enzyme Cre recombinase either under the transcriptional regulation of the glucagon promoter, or under control of the promoter for the GLP-1 receptor. These bespoke Cre-expressing strains can be crossed with commercially available reporter mice which encode fluorescent proteins that are only expressed after removal of lox-stop sequences by Cre. Consequently, one strain (Glu-Cre-RFP) expresses red fluorescent protein (RFP) only in cells where the glucagon promoter is active and the other strain (GLP1R-Cre-RFP) expresses RFP in cells that synthesise GLP-1R. It is important to note however, that since activation of Cre irreversibly turns on RFP expression, all cells where the promoter has been active at any point during development appear fluorescent even if they no longer express GLP-1 or GLP-1R in the adult.

The ability to identify these cells in *ex vivo* tissue has allowed extensive examination of PPG and GLP-1R cells with electrophysiological *in vitro* methods. Perhaps an often overlooked benefit of transgenic systems is to enhance existing immunohistochemical methods. Cytosolic expression of green fluorescent protein (GFP) or YFP presents an antigen that is distributed through the cell and thus staining of the entire cell including axon and full dendritic tree can be achieved. This enables identification of the cells with significantly more precision — particularly important when co-staining with other neurological markers. This approach has permitted highly accurate and extensive analysis of the distribution of PPG neurons and their axons and of cells expressing GLP-1R throughout the CNS. These findings have clearly demonstrated the relationship between the distribution of PPG axons in a variety of different brain regions associated with food intake and their cognate receptor, GLP-1R.

Another significant advantage of mouse models which express Cre is their potential when combined with Cre-dependent viruses, as endogenous CRE expression enables selective "activation" of viruses in defined cell populations (see Fig. 5.2). Although delivery of viruses

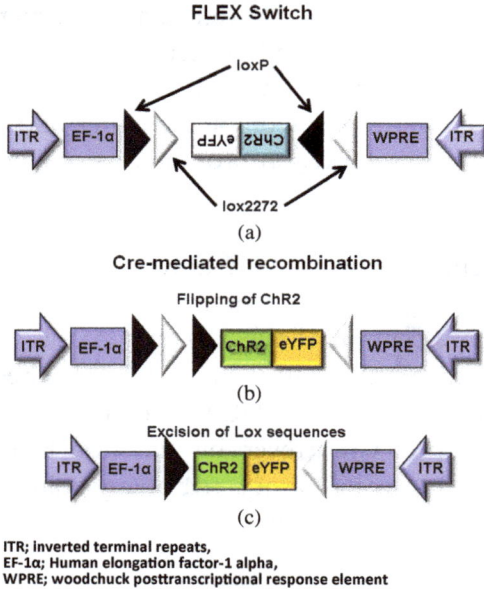

FLEX Switch

(a)

Cre-mediated recombination

Flipping of ChR2

(b)

Excision of Lox sequences

(c)

ITR; inverted terminal repeats,
EF-1α; Human elongation factor-1 alpha,
WPRE; woodchuck posttranscriptional response element

Figure 5.2. FLEX switch activation. (a) the FLEX switch contains two sets of *lox* sequences that flank the ChR2 transgene. ChR2 has been intentionally cloned into the opposite orientation to facilitate expression. The *lox* sequences are heterotypic and anti-parallel and therefore require two Cre-mediated recombination events before stable expression is achieved. (b) Cre inverts the switch, thus inverting the transgene to the correct orientation for expression. (c) the transgene is then locked into place by excision of two *lox* sequences. Only after two recombination events is efficient expression achieved in the presence of Cre.

(discussed in Section 5.3.7) requires surgical procedures, the flexibility of this viral technology allows substantial diversity in the proteins, which can be used to manipulate the cells.

5.3.2. *In vitro Brainstem Slices for Electrophysiology and Imaging*

The brain is very vulnerable to ischemia. When isolating brain tissue, the critical period when damage can occur is from cessation of microvascular blood flow to final maintenance of brainstem slices in oxygenated storage solution. Various precautions, as outlined below, are essential to minimise the impact of the procedure on brain slice quality, imperative for successful experiments.

1. Deeply anaesthetise the adult mouse.
2. Decapitate and submerge the cranium in ice-cold PREP solution (Table 5.1).
3. Extract the brainstem in less than 2 min.
4. Transfer the brainstem to ice-cold PREP solution for 2 min.
5. Place a pre chilled (−20°C) stainless steel heat sink into the vibratome's buffer reservoir.
6. Section to 200 μm thickness in ice-cold PREP solution using a vibratome (5000 mz Campden Instruments Ltd.).

Table 5.1. Solutions for mouse brainstem slice preparation.

	PREP	Recovery	Standard
Temperature (°C)	0–4	30–34	28–34
NaCl (mM)	0	118	118
Sucrose (mM)	200	0	0
KCl (mM)	2.5	3	3
$MgCl_2$ (mM)	7	7	1
$CaCl_2$ (mM)	0.5	0.5	2
$NaHCO_3$ (mM)	28	25	25
NaH_2PO_4 (mM)	1.25	1.2	1.2
D-glucose (mM)	7	2.5	10

(a) For coronal sections place the extracted brainstem on the rostral surface with the cerebellum facing away from the cutting blade.

(b) The PPG neurons are found for a couple of millimeters caudal and rostral from the obex (where the central canal opens into the fourth ventricle).

7. Immediately after cutting, transfer slices to a holding chamber containing 'recovery' solution for 30–60 min at 30–34°C.

8. Transfer slices to "standard" solution for storage up to 10 h at 30–34°C.

- The use of chilled (0–4°C) PREP solution is essential to reduce the electrical activity of the tissue and thus ongoing energy demand during preparation.

- The pH of all solutions is adjusted to 7.4 by constant gassing with carbogen.

Slices need to be contained in a slice-holding chamber heated to 30–34°C. Such a chamber can be constructed as follows: A 50 mL skirted Falcon tube is cut to a height of 5 cm with the conical base removed and replaced with a piece of nylon mesh (200 μm pore size). This chamber is suspended in a 50 mL beaker filled with 25 mL of "standard" solution gassed with carbogen. This enables slices to remain submerged whilst being gassed with carbogen from underneath. The beaker is placed in a block heater to keep it at 30–34°C.

Brainstem slices remain viable for up to 10 hours and are suitable for electrical or optical recordings under a fixed-stage upright microscope using a water immersion lens (usually 40× or 60× magnification) with a working distance of >1 mm to facilitate pipette positioning and equipped with differential interference contrast (DIC) optics. Additionally, an epifluorescence system is required (e.g. a halogen lamp, and excitation plus emission filters specific to the fluorescent label) to identify YFP- or RFP-labelled PPG neurons, or to excite fluorescent dyes.

For experiments, a single brainstem slice is transferred to the recording chamber and held in place by a nylon net fixed to a platinum or tantalum frame (same dimensions as a staple). Superfusate is administered at a flow rate of 5 mL/min and kept at 28–32°C in the recording chamber. Tubing for the superfusion system should be impermeable to gases — in particular oxygen (O_2) and carbon dioxide (CO_2), to ensure that superfusate pO_2 and pH, respectively, do not change during flow to the recording chamber. Stainless steel or Tygon® tubing is recommended for this purpose. For optimal neuronal viability, flow rates should be at least 3–5 mL/min.

5.3.3. *Single-Cell RT-PCR*

The combination of single-cell reverse transcription polymerase chain reaction (RT-PCR) and electrical recordings creates a link between expression of specific proteins and electrical properties of individual cells. At the end of a patch-clamp recording, cytoplasm from the recorded cell is harvested into 6 µL of sterile-filtered pipette solution under visual control. Suction is applied to the patch-clamp electrode and the flow of cytoplasm into the electrode is observed. Successful aspiration of cytoplasm from YFP-expressing cells can be confirmed by green fluorescence inside the electrode. During suction, care has to be taken to maintain the "Gigaseal" between electrode and cell membrane.

1. To synthesise first-strand cDNA from the harvested cytoplasm, expel the 6 μL pipette solution containing cell cytoplasm into an nuclease free 0.5 mL PCR tube.
2. To ensure all harvested cytoplasm is transferred into this solution, crush the electrode tip into the bottom of the tube.
3. Add 4 μL reverse transcription buffer containing 5 µM random hexamer primers, 5 mM dithiothreitol, 0.5 mM dNTPs, 20 U ribonuclease inhibitor and 100 U Superscript III reverse transcriptase (Life Technologies).
4. Incubate for 1 h at 37°C.
5. For PCR amplification of specific gene targets use the cDNA transcribed after step 4 in a PCR reaction as a template with primers specific to each target designed with a Tm around 58°C.
6. To 5 μL of cDNA add 12.5 μL 2X Go-Taq Hot Start Master Mix (Promega), 2.5 μL of 10 mM primer pairs and 5 μL of nuclease-free water.
7. Incubate in a Thermal Cycler using the following conditions: 35 cycles, 30 s at 94°C, 60 s at 58°C, 3 min at 72°C.

8. To increase sensitivity for single cell RT-PCR a second PCR amplification step using nested primers (i.e. primers that target the amplicon synthesised in the first PCR (steps 6 and 7)), is recommended. Instead of cDNA use 2 µL of the first PCR product as a template and repeat steps 6 and 7.

- Negative control reactions should be performed: use H_2O instead of a cDNA sample (water control), solution from pipettes which were inserted into the brainstem slice but without recording from a cell (pipette control), and with samples that have not been reverse transcribed (RT control).
- For positive controls, use a 1:100 dilution of brainstem cDNA.
- Primer pairs should be designed to bind to different exons whenever possible to ensure that PCR products from genomic contamination would be longer than those from mRNA transcripts.

5.3.4. *Brain Tissue Harvest via Transcardial Perfusion*

Perfectly preserved tissue is the most important prerequisite for high quality immunohistochemical or immunofluorescent characterisation of brain tissue. Fast and efficient fixation is best achieved via transcardial perfusion under terminal anesthesia.

1. Deeply anaesthetise mice with an injectable anesthetic (e.g. Pentobarbital; 60 mg/kg; intraperitoneal) to achieve loss of the toe withdrawal reflex.
2. Expose the sternum by making an incision in the skin over the abdomen.
3. Lift the skin over the chest using forceps and extend the incision towards the head to reveal the diaphragm and thorax.
4. Cut open the diaphragm and ribcage to expose the heart.
5. Lift the sternum and clamp towards the head with a surgical needle holder to create a window allowing unobstructed access to the heart. Crucial at this step to avoid excess bleeding.
6. Insert a blunt catheter (18 gauge) into the left ventricle of the heart and clamp in place with a surgical needle holder.
7. Sever the vena cava.

8. Perfuse the animal by slowly injecting 50 mL heparinised phosphate-buffered saline (PBS) to wash out blood.
9. Perfuse with 50 mL phosphate-buffered 4% paraformaldehyde (PB-PFA).
10. Extract the brain and "post-fix" in PB-PFA at 4°C overnight.
11. Incubate the brain in 30% sucrose in PBS to protect the brain tissue from freezing.
12. Cryo-protection is complete once the solution has penetrated the brain causing it to sink to the bottom, usually within 48 h.
13. Embed the tissue in cryomatrix (e.g. OCT (optimum cutting temperature) compound) and section on a cryostat or freezing microtome.
14. We recommend cutting 30-µm-thick free-floating serial brainstem sections for analysis.
15. Store sections in PBS for use in immunofluorescence protocols.

5.3.5. *Immunofluorescent Characterization of Neurons*

For immunofluorescence visualisation of cells expressing YFP (e.g. mGLU Venus mice):

1. Incubate brainstem sections for 30 min in "block" solution (10% goat serum, 1% BSA, 0.3% triton X-100 in PBS).
2. Remove block solution and incubate section with a polyclonal chicken antibody against green fluorescent protein (GFP; 1:1500; Abcam) diluted in block solution at 4°C.
3. Remove polyclonal antibody and wash 5 times with PBS.
4. Incubate sections with a goat anti-chicken IgG AlexaFluor488 conjugate (1:500; Invitrogen) in the dark for 2 h at room temperature.
5. Wash sections again as in step 3.
6. Arrange sections on a glass microscope slide using a fine paintbrush and leave to air dry, protecting from dust.
7. Once dried add a couple of drops of an aqueous mounting compound, e.g. Vectashield (Vector Laboratories; www.vectorlabs.com), and gently place a coverslip on top.

8. Store slices at 4°C until ready for analysis using a fluorescence microscope.

• This basic protocol can easily be adapted for a variety of different primary and secondary antibodies. In each case the optimal dilution has to be determined empirically and the block solution needs to be adjusted based on the secondary antibody used. For example, to visualise catecholaminergic cells with a polyclonal rabbit antibody raised against tyrosine-hydroxylase (anti-TH, 1:500; Santa Cruz) the block solution contains 10% sheep serum and a sheep anti-rabbit IgG CY-3 conjugate (1:500; Sigma) secondary antibody is used.

5.3.6. *Functional Manipulation of the GLP-1 System*

The most widely used experimental approach to manipulating the brain GLP-1 system has been the administration of exogenous GLP-1, GLP-1 agonists or GLP-1 antagonists either via i.c.v. infusion or more recently via targeted injection into various brain nuclei to look for direct effects caused by receptor activation or blockade (for review see[8]). Injection of GLP-1R antagonists in satiated animals has demonstrated a physiological role for endogenous GLP-1 in the brain. Dissecting the specific neuronal populations involved in these processes is impossible using i.c.v. infusion. However, combining specific viral vector approaches and precise stereotaxic injection will allow more appropriate physiological activation and, crucially, the separation from pan-CNS receptor activation.

Stereotaxic injection is not a trivial procedure. The complexity of intricate recovery surgery on small rodents requires expertise to ensure humane and refined experiments can be conducted. Most commonly, injection targets are located in the forebrain. These require a cranial window to be drilled into the skull to allow the injection pipettes to penetrate into the cerebrum. To ensure targeting of the desired area, a brain atlas for the specific species is necessary to determine the appropriate coordinates. These are universally applicable and derived in relation to two key landmarks on the skull; bregma and lambda. For injections into the brainstem, an alternative procedure is required where dissection through the semispinalis capitis and underlying muscles reveals the anterior atlantooccipital membrane. The membrane requires delicate puncturing to reveal the underlying brainstem at the location of the calamus scriptorius, from which point injection coordinates are determined.

5.3.7. *Molecular Targeting of the PPG Neurons*

Global knockouts of the GLP-1 receptor or PPG have yielded little insight into the role of GLP-1-mediated signalling. This might be due to compensatory mechanisms acting during development. To overcome such problems when assessing the precise role of GLP-1-producing neurons, it is imperative to (a) selectively target these cells in a fully developed adult animal, (b) target specific populations of GLP-1-expressing cells whilst leaving the others intact (Table 5.2), and (c) control the temporal pattern of the activation or inactivation of these cells. Such a possibility is particularly important in light of the fact that feeding state and/or circadian rhythm are likely to modulate physiological effects evoked by activation of these cells.

Specific targeting of the PPG neurons has been achieved by precise stereotaxic injection into the NTS of lentiviruses designed to knock down expression of GLP-1 using RNA interference.[9] Whilst this method achieved a 50% reduction of PPG mRNA, a substantial proportion of endogenous mRNA was still present. The capacity of this method to fully reduce expression in PPG terminals located in the PVN was less effective, achieving only a 30% decrease. Expanding the use of the glucagon promoter to enable cell-specific expression of virally encoded genes will likely prove difficult due to the uncharacterised nature of the putative promoter region. Also, due to the nature of viral vectors only a limited amount of nucleic acid can be incorporated into each viral particle (Table 5.3). As promoters are often large and not easily defined linear sections of DNA, the limited capacity of the viral particle prevents their usage.

Targeting the desired population of cells in the CNS requires logical planning (Fig. 5.4). A combination of precise spatial targeting via stereotaxic injection, combined with a selective viral system ensures specificity (Table 5.3 and Fig. 5.3). There are several avenues

Table 5.2.   Types of promoters to regulate gene expression.

Promoter type	Constitutive	Cell-type-specific	Inducible	Synthetic (bespoke specificity)
Specificity	Non-specific, widely expressed, functions across most tissue types. Requires combining with another method (e.g. Cre expression) to achieve selectivity. Elicits high levels of transgene expression.	Controls transcription in selective tissues, or during specific developmental stages. Can be used cross-species.	Requires environmental triggers to facilitate expression, which can be highly controlled. Triggers include: light, antibiotics, steroids etc.	Artificially constructed from multiple repeating regions of DNA sequences, which normally bind to cell-type-specific transcription factors.
Examples	**Chicken-Beta actin CMV** (Cytomegalovirus)	**GFAP** (glial fibrillary acidic protein) promoter: specific to astrocytes; **Synapsin** promoter: Specific to neurons; **GAD65** (glutamate decarboxylase) promoter: specific for GABAergic neurons.	**Tet-on/Tet-off** system: requires doxycycline to promote expression of transgene.	**PRSx8**: specifically binds the endogenous transcription factor Phox2B in autonomic neurons.

Table 5.3. Viral vectors as neuroscientific tools.

Virus	Adenovirus (Adv)	Lentivirus (LV)	Adeno-associated virus (AAV)
Genome and particle size	dsDNA, 90–100 nm diameter, non-enveloped.	ssRNA, 80–100 nm diameter, enveloped.	dsDNA, 20–25 nm diameter, non-enveloped.
Coding capacity	Up to ~8 Kb for standard vectors, ~30 kb for "gutless".	Up to ~12 Kb	Up to ~4.7 Kb
Production	New viral constructs require co-transfection of DNA plasmids to form nascent virus particles. Once formed, particles can be amplified using HEK293 cells. Large-scale amplification to achieve high titres takes weeks. Advs can be purified from lysed cells using Caesium chloride (CsCl) gradient ultracentrifugation or commercial kits.	Viral particles are formed by co-transfection of DNA plasmids (three or four plasmids, for second or third generation system respectively). Viral particles are collected in supernatant and can be purified using ultracentrifugation. Production time 3–4 days.	AAVs are naturally incapable of self-replication. They require infection from other viruses (adenovirus, herpes simplex virus) to replicate. Formation of viruses *in vitro* requires transfection of DNA plasmids into HEK2893 cells. Particles can be purified using heparin columns for serotype 2 or via CsCl gradient for others.
Expression	From 12 h to 14 d. Expression is transient as viral genome doesn't integrate; genome exists as an episome.	Stable expression can be observed from around 21 d and can last for months. Some LVs can integrate into the host genome; others (integration defective) exist as an episome.	Stable expression can be observed from around 21 d and can persist for months. Viral genome exists stably as an episome.

(Continued)

Table 5.3. (*Continued*)

Virus	Adenovirus (Adv)	Lentivirus (LV)	Adeno-associated virus (AAV)
Tropism	Infects glia, neurons and other brain cells. In some neurons can move in a retrograde direction.	Require pseudo-typing with Vesicular stomatitis virus-glycoproteins for stability and tropism. VSV-G-coated LVs do not move in a retrograde direction. Infects dividing and non-dividing cells, but prefers neurons.	No immune response; used in human clinical trials. Specificity of cells is determined by serotypes. AAV-2 is most commonly used for CNS.
Advantages and disadvantages	Genome cannot integrate so expression of transgenes doesn't persist. Good for organotypic culture (*ex vivo*) infection. Elicits an immune response.	Insertional mutagenesis can raise potential safety questions depending on the 2nd or 3rd helper system; possible germ line alterations. Tropism can be altered via different pseudo-typing. No immuonogenic proteins.	Low coding capacity. Requires transfection and purification for each batch, takes approximately 10 d as it does not replicate. Elicits a very low immune response.

Synthesis of purified recombinant viruses for *in vitro* or *in vivo* applications

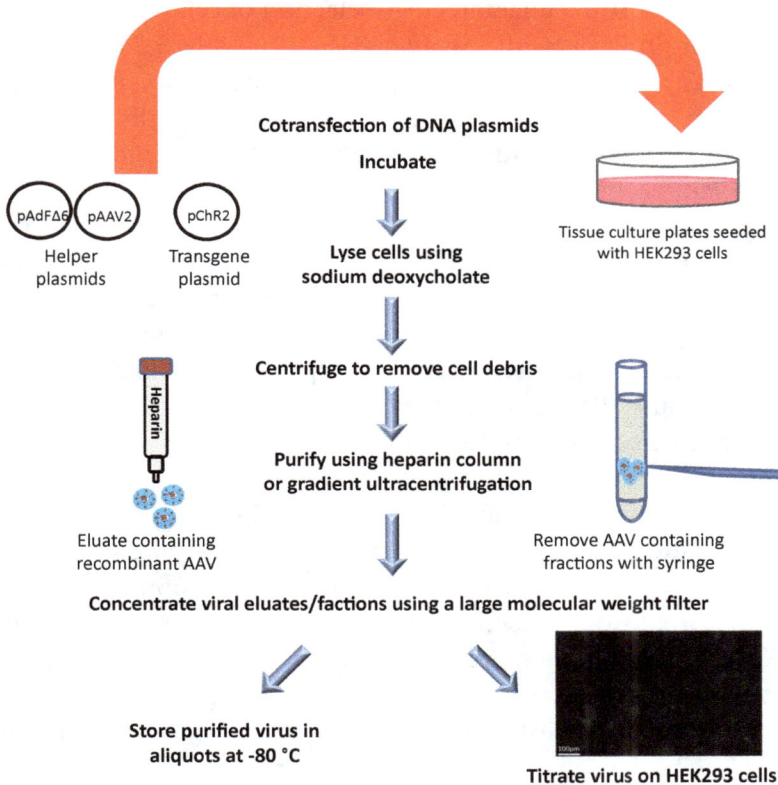

Figure 5.3. Production of recombinant AAVs expressing a transgene ChannelRhodopsin2 (ChR2). Nascent virus particles are formed by co-transfection of DNA plasmids encoding the transgene flanked by inverted terminal repeats specific to the AAV serotype of choice and helper plasmids expressing adenoviral proteins (pAdFΔ6) and the specific serotype replicase and capsid proteins (e.g. pAAV2). After 72 h, cells are lysed and nucleic acids are digested using the mild detergent sodium deoxycholate and benzonase endonuclease for 1 h at 37°C. Cell debris is removed by centrifugation at 300g for 15 min prior to purification. Serotype 2 AAVs are loaded into a heparin column and eluted with increasing concentrations of NaCl. All other serotypes are added to a caesium chloride or iodixional gradient prior to ultracentrifugation. Purified viruses can be stored at −80°C. Titrate viruses on HEK293 cells — viral titre can be determined after 72 h by counting cells expressing the fluorescent reporter protein.

to achieve expression that is limited to the correct cell type. A popular choice employs the use of tissue-specific promoters that allow a high — but not 100%-guaranteed — selection of cell type. Promoters such as glial fibrillary acidic protein (GFAP) (Table 5.2) permit targeting of astrocytes, whereas synapsin facilitates expression in neurons. Such promoters make tissue-specific targeting of small populations difficult because of viral diffusion. To combat this, the development of bespoke artificial promoters such as PRSx8, which only permits transgene expression in cells containing the transcription factor PHOX2B (Table 5.2), can improve specificity. A significant drawback is that artificial promoters are difficult to make and obtaining a promoter for each cell type is difficult. Even with the use of tissue-specific promoters, limiting expression to highly distinct populations like the PPG neurons is impossible. In such instances further specificity is required and often requires a transgenic approach employing Cre (as discussed in Section 5.3.1) to activate viruses inside the desired cell population. This strategy selectively involves the combination of the available transgenic mouse strains that express Cre and Cre-dependent viruses, where gene expression is controlled either by a lox "stop" cassette or the more stringent recently created FLEX switch system (Fig. 5.2). In particular, the stringency achieved with the FLEX switch system is superior to that of a lox "stop" cassette, which can exhibit low levels of expression even in the absence of Cre. Furthermore, using either Cre-dependent viral system allows the use of strong, constitutive promoters.

The combinations of viruses with different promoters that can encode a plethora of desired transgenes are almost limitless. Optogenes are routinely delivered to target cells using viral vectors, as are intracellular fluorescent sensors like GCaMP, Perceval, and eCALWY. G-protein-coupled receptors like DREADDs, which only respond to inert exogenous ligands delivered by injection or through drinking water, can also be expressed in this way. The significant advantages of engineering viral vectors is that once constructed they are transferable to different animal models and to various tissue locations, and it is easy to amplify production.

5.3.8. *The Importance of Timing*

GLP-1 release in the gut is post-prandial, and most meals are ingested during the more active parts of the day. Whether investigating rodent models or directly observing humans, it is crucial to determine the most appropriate time to study the physiological role of the PPG neurons. Rodents are usually more active after sunset and ingest more of their food during this period. This is in direct contrast to humans. But the role of GLP-1 in the CNS might operate on an entirely different time scale to the two-minute half-life of that in the gut. Therefore determining the precise time when PPG neurons should be active is difficult. There is evidence that suggests a distinct difference in their ability to sense stimuli depending on the time of day. In fact, targeting of the NAc core with the GLP-1 receptor antagonist Ex9 has been shown to increase food intake most effectively up to two hours after animals have entered the dark phase of the circadian cycle. This suggests that the sensitivity of GLP-1-mediated satiety driven by the PPG neurons does not occur throughout the entirety of the 24-hour day.

However, the circadian cycle is not the only temporal consideration. Evidence has shown that GLP-1-mediated effects are far more pronounced directly after a meal. It has long been demonstrated that i.c.v. injection of GLP-1 greatly reduces food intake, but injection of the GLP-1R antagonist Ex9 strongly increased food intake and body weight in satiated animals only, not in fasted rats. This crucial demonstration shows that endogenous GLP-1 release also varies with the animal's feeding state.

It is therefore a significant challenge to determine when animals are in the correct feeding state so that false negative results can be avoided. Elucidating this in relation to the circadian rhythm of PPG neuronal activation has not been determined and clearly meal times as well as the circadian cycle have to be considered. This also raises further questions when comparing the rodent model with humans, which are strictly diurnal.

5.4. Key Challenges

Investigations of the central GLP-1 system are commonly approached from two different angles. On one hand, research aims to uncover the role of endogenous GLP-1 in the control of body homeostasis; on the other hand, the increasing use of GLP-1 analogues in the treatment of T2D has prompted research into prevention of adverse effects associated with drugs such as liraglutide and exenatide. One approach is motivated by the desire to understand basic physiology, whereas the other is based on supraphysiological activation of the GLP-1 system. However, many of the essential questions are the same.

5.4.1. *GLP-1R Distribution and Function*

Due to the lack of sufficiently specific antibodies, the distribution of GLP-1R in the brain has been investigated using binding assays with labelled GLP-1 and *in situ* hybridisation. Recently, however, a transgenic mouse model has been developed, which may provide new insight into the distribution and function of GLP-1R expressing cells. As described in Section 5.3, the GLP-1R-Cre-RFP mouse model co-expresses Cre and tdRFP in GLP-1R cells.[10] Using this mouse model, GLP-1R-positive cells have already been identified in areas of the brainstem, hypothalamus, and vagus nerve. However, the distribution in the rest of the brain has not been described. Furthermore, the characteristics of the GLP-1R cells are unexplored. Using the transgenic mouse model described above, the following questions could be addressed:

- Firstly, which cell types express GLP-1R in different areas of the brain and which neurotransmitters are co-expressed? This can be investigated by immunohistological co-staining for RFP and various neurotransmitters or cell-type-specific markers, such as GAD65/67 (for GABAergic), tyrosine hydroxylase (for catecholaminergic), ChAT (cholinergic), VGluT1/2 (glutamatergic), or 5-HT transporter (serotonergic). The same immunohistological approach can also be used to map the projection targets of the GLP-1R neurons.
- Secondly, what are the electrophysiological properties of the GLP-1R cells and which non-GLP-1 stimuli do they respond to?

This question can be answered by performing patch-clamp recordings on RFP-positive cells.

• Finally, what is the physiological role of different populations of GLP-1R-expressing neurons? This last question relies on the molecular handle provided by the expression of Cre recombinase in these cells. By injecting a Cre-dependent viral vector as described in Section 5.3, the populations of GLP-1R cells in distinct brain regions can be either activated or inhibited while monitoring physiological parameters such as blood glucose, food intake, body temperature, heart rate, and blood pressure in live animals.

5.4.2. *The role of Endogenously Produced Central GLP-1*

Although plenty of evidence supports a role for GLP-1 receptors expressed in the brain, the role of the GLP-1-producing neurons remains more obscure and it has yet to be proven unequivocally that PPG neurons release GLP-1. Most studies investigating the role of central GLP-1 have injected supraphysiological doses of GLP-1 or its analogues. This raises the question whether the results are truly representative of endogenous GLP-1 release from hindbrain PPG neurons. Different approaches could be taken to answer this question with the Glu-Cre-RFP transgenic mouse as an essential tool (see Section 5.3). Cre-dependent viral vectors could be used to ablate PPG neurons and thus abolish the endogenous source of GLP-1 in the brain, and the effects on physiological outputs monitored. Importantly, the feeding status of the animal has been shown to affect the outcome of GLP-1R activation, prompting caution when planning and interpreting experiments. Furthermore, the projection targets of PPG neurons range from cardiovascular control centres via nuclei regulating energy balance to the mesolimbic reward pathways. It will therefore be exciting to see whether distinct subpopulations of PPG neurons control distinct brain areas and whether these subpopulations respond to different stimuli. Since the location of the subpopulations is the only distinguishing factor, only the stereotactic injection of Cre-dependent viral vectors into Glu-Cre-RFP transgenic mice provides the necessary accuracy. Finally, the development of tools for monitoring

Incretin Biology — A Practical Guide

and manipulating whole-animal physiology enables investigations of the role of the central GLP-1 system in conscious, live animals. By combining techniques such as telemetry and virally mediated transgene expression, the PPG neurons (Fig. 5.4) can be either inhibited or

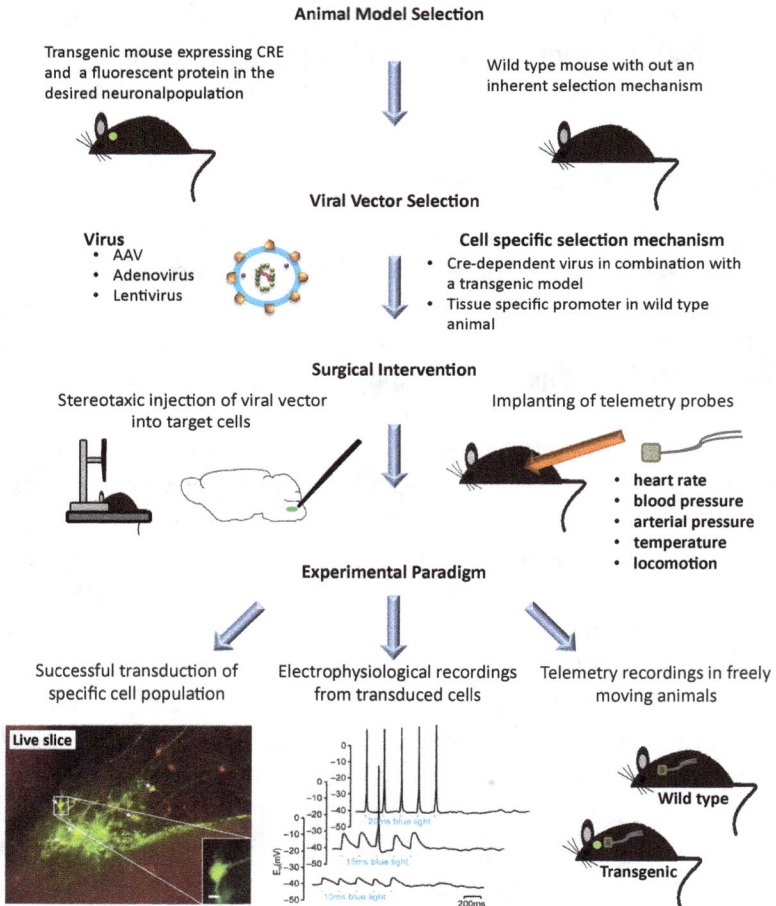

Experimental strategy to target a specific neuronal population in the CNS

Animal Model Selection

Transgenic mouse expressing CRE and a fluorescent protein in the desired neuronalpopulation

Wild type mouse with out an inherent selection mechanism

Viral Vector Selection

Virus
- AAV
- Adenovirus
- Lentivirus

Cell specific selection mechanism
- Cre-dependent virus in combination with a transgenic model
- Tissue specific promoter in wild type animal

Surgical Intervention

Stereotaxic injection of viral vector into target cells

Implanting of telemetry probes

- heart rate
- blood pressure
- arterial pressure
- temperature
- locomotion

Experimental Paradigm

Successful transduction of specific cell population

Electrophysiological recordings from transduced cells

Telemetry recordings in freely moving animals

Live slice

Wild type

Transgenic

Figure 5.4.   Overview of strategy for selective neuronal targeting using a selective viral technology allowing multiple stage investigation in acute slice and freely moving animals. Surgical intervention requires stereotaxic injection of a viral vector to transduce cells in a mouse model. Optional additional surgery can be performed to examine

Figure 5.4. (*Continue on facing page*) the effects of virally expressed transgenes using telemetry probes that are capable of recording and transmitting a variety of physiological outputs. Experimental paradigm: selective viral transduction of PPG neurons (red) with high-level expression of ChR2:eYFP in the NTS (inset scale bar 10 μm). Electrical activity of PPG neurons expressing ChR2 in acute slices analysed with whole-cell patch-clamp recordings. In current clamp, laser light stimulation at 455 nm of 20 ms duration reliably elicited action potentials in PPG neurons, shorter light pulses (10–20 ms) caused smaller depolarisations and decreased probability of eliciting action potentials. Blue bars indicate light stimulation.

activated while monitoring the effect on a range of physiological and behavioural parameters.

5.4.3. *Brain and Periphery — Two Systems, One Goal?*

The discovery that GLP-1 not only acts as an incretin but also has powerful effects on the CNS prompts two questions. Firstly, do the central and peripheral GLP-1 systems work together or do they function as separate entities with distinct functions? Secondly, what is the link, if any, between these two systems? Evidence based on peripheral injections of GLP-1R agonists or antagonists suggests that GLP-1 in the bloodstream activates central circuits. However, the pathway leading to this activation remains under debate. In one simple model, GLP-1 released from the L cells in the gut reaches GLP-1Rs in the areas of the brain not protected by the BBB, the circumventricular organs. Neurons in these areas would then relay the signal to other parts of the brain. However, the short half-life of GLP-1 in the bloodstream makes it unlikely that the endogenous peptide released from L cells will reach receptors in the circumventricular organs. GLP-1 analogues, however, which are less susceptible to degradation by DPP-IV, may be able to activate such receptors. This again demonstrates the need for careful dissection of the differences between supraphysiological and endogenous activation of the central GLP-1 system.

An alternative model proposes that GLP-1 activates receptors expressed on the vagus nerve close to the site of release in the gut. In this model, vagal afferents expressing GLP-1R are activated by GLP-1 released nearby and transmit an electrical signal to the brainstem via the solitary tract. Intriguingly, electrical stimulation of the solitary tract activates NTS PPG neurons, providing a possible link between peripheral release of GLP-1 in response to food intake and activation of central GLP-1 receptors.

The involvement of each proposed pathway in relaying a peripheral GLP-1 signal to the PPG neurons could be investigated by injecting GLP-1 peripherally while monitoring the activity of the PPG neurons in the live animal. Selective deafferentation of the vagus nerve would reveal any involvement of the vagus nerve, whereas knockdown of GLP-1Rs in the circumventricular organs using Cre-dependent viral vector would uncover the role of these brain areas. By using both GLP-1 and liraglutide or Ex4 in independent experiments, the differences in their actions could be investigated.

5.4.4. *Adverse Effects of GLP-1 Analogues*

GLP-1 analogues used as treatment for T2D have side effects in humans, many of which can be attributed to effects on the CNS. These include nausea, headaches, diarrhoea, reduced appetite, and possibly tachycardia. As mentioned previously, GLP-1 analogues are given in supraphysiological doses and are less susceptible to degradation by DPP-IV than the endogenous peptide. Any adverse effects on the CNS may therefore not represent true functions of the endogenous system but may be a result of over-activation of GLP-1R. There is a demand for dissection of the mechanisms behind these secondary effects, whether unwanted or desirable (i.e. nausea versus weight loss). Understanding the pathways responsible for each effect will facilitate development of drugs with minimal unwanted side effects. Since most investigations use rodent models, a logical question is: how conserved is the central GLP-1 system between humans and rodents? GLP-1-expressing neurons are located in the same areas of humans and rodents. The next important step will be to map the projections of the GLP-1 expressing neurons in humans and compare with the rodent models. Since side effects of GLP-1 analogues in humans and rodents are largely similar, it is expected that the distribution of GLP-1 receptor and PPG neuronal projections are comparable in rodents and humans.

5.5. Conclusions

- GLP-1 receptors in the CNS contribute to the anorexic and hypo-glycaemic effects of systemically administered GLP-1.
- Stereotaxic injection of GLP-1 or its analogues into specific brain nuclei has pinpointed different GLP-1 effects to distinct brain regions.
- Stereotaxic injection of GLP-1R antagonists has demonstrated a physiological role for endogenous GLP-1 in the brain.
- Some clinically observed side effects of GLP-1 analogues might involve activation of the central GLP-1 system; identifying the exact pathways could help to develop stategies to reduce these effects.
- Transgenic mouse models allow for specific identification of PPG neurones and GLP-1R-expressing cells.
- Direct control of PPG neuron function *in vivo* will provide the next important step in dissecting the role of brain GLP-1.
- Elucidating the exact function of the central GLP-1 system and its interaction with peripherally released GLP-1 in an animal model remain key challenges for the near future.

References

1. Vrang, N. and Grove K. (2011). The brainstem preproglucagon system in a non-human primate (Macaca mulatta), *Brain Res.*, **1397**, 28–37.
2. Zheng, H., Cai, L. and Rinaman, L. (2015). Distribution of glucagon-like peptide 1-immunopositive neurons in human caudal medulla, *Brain Struct. Funct.*, **220**, 1213–1219.
3. Llewellyn-Smith, I.J., Reimann, F., Gribble, F.M. and Trapp, S. (2011). Preproglucagon neurons project widely to autonomic control areas in the mouse brain, *Neuroscience*, **180**, 111–121.
4. Llewellyn-Smith, I.J., Marina, N., Manton, R.N., Reimann, F., Gribble, F.M. and Trapp, S. (2015) Spinally projecting preproglucagon axons preferentially innervate sympathetic preganglionic neurons, *Neuroscience*, **284**, 872–887.
5. Beiroa, D., Imbernon, M., Gallego, R., Senra, A., Herranz, D., Villarroya, F., Serrano, M., Fernø, J., Salvador, J., Escalada, J., Dieguez, C., Lopez, M.,

Frühbeck, G. and Nogueiras, R. (2014). GLP-1 agonism stimulates brown adipose tissue thermogenesis and browning through hypothalamic AMPK, *Diabetes*, **63**(10), 3346–3358.

6. Sivertsen, J., Rosenmeier, J., Holst, J.J. and Vilsbøll, T. (2012). The effect of glucagon-like peptide 1 on cardiovascular risk, *Nat. Rev. Cardiol.*, **9**(4), 209–222.

7. Reimann, F., Habib, A.M., Tolhurst, G., Parker, H.E., Rogers, G.J. and Gribble, F.M. (2008). Glucose sensing in L cells: a primary cell study, *Cell Metab.*, **8**(6), 532–539.

8. Trapp, S. and Richards, J.E. (2013). The gut hormone glucagon-like peptide-1 produced in brain: is this physiologically relevant?, *Curr. Opin. Pharmacol.*, **13**(6), 964–969.

9. Barrera, J.G., Jones, K.R., Herman, J.P., D'Alessio, D.A., Woods, S.C. and Seeley, R.J. (2011). Hyperphagia and increased fat accumulation in two models of chronic CNS glucagon-like peptide-1 loss of function, *J. Neurosci.*, **31**(10), 3904–3913.

10. Richards, P., Parker, H.E., Adriaenssens, A.E., Hodgson, J.M., Cork, S.C., Trapp, S., Gribble, F.M. and Reimann, F. (2014). Identification and characterization of GLP-1 receptor-expressing cells using a new transgenic mouse model, *Diabetes*, **63**(4), 1224–1233.

Chapter 6

Bariatric Surgery: Clinical Aspects

C. Tsironis and A. Ahmed

Department of Surgery, Imperial College London

6.1. Introduction

Behavioural and pharmacological treatments of morbid obesity may lead to short-term total body weight loss of around 5%; however, they cannot fully resolve obesity-related comorbidities, nor show long-term sustained success. Bariatric surgery is the most effective treatment of morbid obesity as it results in long-term sustained weight loss and remission of comorbidities.

The history of obesity surgery dates back to the 1950s with the Swedish surgeon Viktor Henrikson, who performed a massive small bowel resection in order to create a short bowel to aid with weight loss. After this attempt, various other surgeons performed similar small bowel bypasses. The jejunoileal bypass (JIB) had satisfactory weight loss results; it led to malabsorption by bypassing most of the intestine while keeping the stomach intact. However, eventually the procedure was found to be associated with serious complications.

The gastric bypass was developed by Edward Mason in the 1960s. The basis for this surgery was that patients undergoing partial gastrectomy for ulcers concomitantly lost weight. The gastric bypass consisted of dissecting the stomach across the horizontal axis and constructing a gastrojejunal loop bypass. This procedure was associated with bile reflux. This procedure was modified by Griffen, who performed it as a "Roux-en-Y" with a limb of intestine anastomosed to a gastric pouch, so that bile would not pass through the stomach. The operation was further modified by Torres, who presented the vertical pouch on the lesser curvature of the stomach. Many modifications have followed since then. The first case series of laparoscopic Roux-en-Y gastric bypass (RYGB) was reported by Wittgrove and Clark in 1994.

While the bypass was being developed, another operation, the biliopancreatic diversion (BPD), was introduced by Scopinaro. This procedure causes controlled malabsorption; it only permits absorption in the distal 50–70 cm of the ileum and this has fewer side effects than the JIB. The duodenal switch (DS) was a modification of the BPD developed by Hess to prevent some of the complications of the latter and consists of a sleeve gastrectomy associated with a duodenoenterostomy. Vertical sleeve gastrectomy (VSG), often performed as a sole initial operation, has the option to add the DS or RYGB as a second operation if there is insufficient weight loss or if indeed there is weight regain.

Also in the 1970s, gastroplasty was an alternative to the RYGB and the JIB. In 1982 Mason described the vertical banded gastroplasty (VBG), in which a vertical pouch is fashioned along the lesser curve of the stomach with the outlet controlled by a non-dilatable band.

Gastric banding, which is still a popular procedure to date, was introduced in the 1980s by Molina as another restrictive procedure. A number of non-surgical procedures have also been developed as a treatment for excess weight, including the intragastric balloon and the EndoBarrier Gastrointestinal Liner System.

Surgical treatment of obesity results in sustained weight loss, benefits patients with obesity-related comorbidities and also reduces relative risk of death. Thus the demand for bariatric surgery has risen dramatically in recent years. There are various clinical indications for surgical intervention based on the US National Institutes of Health criteria (Table 6.1).

Table 6.1.   Eligibility criteria for surgical intervention for treatment of obesity.

Body mass index (BMI) $\geq 40\,\mathrm{kg/m^2}$.*

BMI $\geq 35\ \mathrm{kg/m^2}$ and obesity-related comorbidities (T2DM, OSA, or joint issues).

Patient has followed all other methods for weight loss (exercise, diet, medication), including six-month medically supervised program, but has not been able to sustain weight loss.

No specific medical or psychological reasons for not undergoing the operation.

Patient fit enough to undergo an anaesthetic and operation.

Understanding of the need for long-term follow-up.

* In the UK, the National Institute for Clinical Excellence recommends that patients with BMI ≥ 50 should be considered directly for surgery without the need for a prior six-month medically supervised weight loss.

6.2. Surgical Procedures for the Treatment of Obesity

The following sections provide detailed instructions for use by qualified surgeons embarking on bariatric surgery in man.

6.2.1. *Laparoscopic Adjustable Gastric Band*

Laparoscopic adjustable gastric band (LAGB) insertion begins with the creation of a pneumoperitoneum (Fig. 6.1(a)). The left lobe of the liver is retracted and investigation for presence of hiatus hernia takes place. If a hiatus hernia is recognized it should be repaired before the insertion of the band. The standard approach takes place through a retrogastric window between the pas flaccida medially and the angle of His laterally, as this reduces the risk of band slippage. The band should be checked and prepared according to the instructions of the manufacturer before inserting it in the abdominal cavity. The band is slipped through into the correct position and closed to create a small "virtual" gastric pouch. Three or four sutures should be used to plicate the stomach over the anterior surface of the band in order to keep it in place and prevent slippage. The band is connected via a tube to a port reservoir. The latter is placed in the subcutaneous layer of the anterior abdominal wall over the rectus fascia, so that the band can be adjusted in an outpatient setting to reach the optimal restriction. The operation takes place as a day case and lasts approximately 30–40 min.

In the past, gastric banding was considered to work as a purely restrictive mechanism. According to O'Brien *et al.*, restriction is not directly related to weight loss.[1] Approximately 70% of patients experience elimination of hunger following gastric band insertion. Pressure applied on the vagus nerve by the band is considered to be the predominant hypothesis to explain the decreased hunger after gastric banding.[1] Peptide YY (PYY), glucagon-like peptide 1 (GLP-1) and oxyntomodulin (OXM) do not seem to play a role.

The adjustable gastric band is the safest among the surgical interventions for treatment of obesity, with an operative mortality of less than 0.1%. On the other hand there is a 5–10% risk for reoperation over the following 10 years due to complications related to the initial procedure.

The complications after gastric band insertion can be related either to the band itself or to the port. The band-related complications include band slippage 4%, erosion of the gastric wall 1%, pouch or oesophageal dilation 5–10%, gastric perforation 0.1% and obstruction of the gastric lumen. The incidence of port-related complications is 5–10% in total and includes infection of the abdominal wall around the port, port displacement and needle-stick injury to the tube of the port.

Gastric band slippage occurs when the stomach below the band herniates above it. In this situation excessive gastric tissue is trapped inside the band resulting in obstruction of the gastric lumen between the pouch above the band and the stomach below. The patient usually presents with nausea and vomiting. On the other hand, gastric band erosion consists of gradual intrusion of the band into the gastric lumen, and sometimes the whole band may end up inside the stomach. The clinical presentation includes weight regain and port infection. The risk of gastric or oesophageal perforation is very low and is due to intraoperative dissection during the band implantation. Another complication of the procedure is gastric pouch and oesophageal dilation. The former occurs as symmetrical enlargement of the gastric pouch above the band, which may in turn result in dilation and malfunction of the oesophagus. This condition is usually a result of an over-filled band and/or of excessive eating. The patients present with symptoms of reflux as well as reduced satiety, but it is not usually associated with obstructive symptoms. The above complication may be managed conservatively by temporarily de-filling the band, but surgical intervention and removal of the band may be needed in some cases. Obstruction of the gastric lumen between the upper and lower part of the stomach can occur either in the early postoperative period as a result of oedema or haematoma around the band, or afterwards due to lack of compliance with the appropriate diet and bolus obstruction.

The efficacy of the gastric banding on weight loss depends very much on the unit that performs it and on patient compliance with follow-up. Most units report approximately 20% of total body weight loss. According to data reported by some Australian units, approximately 30% of total weight loss may be achieved with adjustable gastric banding.

6.2.2. *Roux-en-Y Gastric Bypass*

The RYGB procedure begins with creation of pneumoperitoneum (Fig. 6.1(b)). The liver is retracted, the angle of His is dissected, the lesser sac is entered through the lesser curve and the retrogastric adhesions are freed. A 15–20 mL vertical gastric pouch is created by the application of an endostapler. The operation is continued with identification of the ligament of Treitz and division of the jejunum 40–60 cm distally. The distal part of the jejunum is then moved cephalad and anastomosed to the gastric pouch in order to create the Roux limb or alimentary limb. The gastrojejunostomy can be ante-colic or retro-colic, and ante-gastric or retro-gastric, and can be performed by the application of linear or circular staples or hand-sewn. The proximal part of the jejunum, the biliopancreatic limb, is joined to the Roux limb approximately 100 cm distal to the gastrojejunostomy. The length of the alimentary limb during RYGB has been discussed in several articles. No benefit was found for patients with a BMI of $50 \, \text{kg/m}^2$ or less whose alimentary limb was longer than 150 cm. Alimentary limbs longer than 250 cm resulted in increased weight loss in patients with a BMI greater than $50 \, \text{kg/m}^2$ in comparison with the standard RYGB, but increased nutritional deficiencies and high rate of reoperation were reported for patients whose alimentary limb was longer than 300 cm. The operating time for gastric bypass ranges from 60 min to 90 min and the patient needs to stay as an inpatient for one to two days.

The complications after RYGB include those associated with the bypass and the general complications after bariatric surgery, which may occur after any bariatric operation. The complications related to the procedure itself are bowel obstruction, gastric remnant distention, anastomotic ulcer, bleeding, leak, sepsis, and death. The incidence of bleeding from the anastomoses or the staple lines is 1–2% in the early postoperative period. The risk of leak from the staple lines or the anastomoses is 1–2% and urgent reoperation is required in order to avoid delay in the treatment, which may lead to severe sepsis and death. The clinical presentation of a leak in the bariatric patient may be mild and if there is any suspicion of leak the bariatric surgeon must be vigilant and consider early reoperation.

Bowel obstruction at the level of the gastrojejunostomy can occur either as a result of a stricture (1%) or due to bolus obstruction. Other causes of small bowel obstruction include internal hernia formation (1–2%). In these cases small bowel loops incarcerate through the mesentery defects of the small bowel or transverse colon. Alimentary limb obstruction can occur if the transverse mesocolic defect is narrow in patients undergoing retrocolic anastomosis. Small bowel obstruction can also occur due to obstruction at the jejunojejunostomy from kinking, stricture, haematoma or blood clot, as well as intussusception, adhesions, and port site hernias.

The risk for developing marginal ulcers after the operation may be up to 5–10%. The causative factors include gastric acid, non-steroidal anti-inflammatory drugs, use of tobacco, *Helicobacter pylori*, gastro–gastric fistula, ischemia and tension of the anastomosis, foreign body (suture), and large gastric pouch.

Other general complications related to all bariatric procedures include venous thromboembolic disease such as deep venous thrombosis (1%) and pulmonary embolism (0.1%). According to the International Bariatric Surgery Registry, the above phenomena represent the most frequent cause of mortality following bariatric surgery; thus, prophylactic measures should be taken against these by using low-molecular-weight heparin, an IVC filter prior to surgery if it is necessary, and calf compression devices, as well as encouraging early mobilisation after surgery. The nutritional complications after surgery can be avoided as long as the patients are compliant with their intake of multivitamin and mineral supplements and attend their follow-up. Blood tests should be taken to screen for iron, calcium and Vitamin D deficiency. Patients who undergo bariatric surgery are at a higher risk of developing gallstones due to rapid weight loss, and may present with symptoms and complications of gallstones such as biliary colic, acute cholecystitis, choledocholithiasis and pancreatitis.

The current thinking regarding mechanisms of action of the RYGB is not related to calorie malabsorption or restriction of food through the gastric pouch. The small volume gastric pouch, the bypass of the remnant stomach and first part of the small bowel, the presence of undiluted bile flow in the first part of the small bowel, the early contact of the mid-jejunum with food and the disruption of the small vagal fibres when the gastric pouch is separated from the gastric remnant are at least five components of the procedure which are considered to contribute to the mechanisms of weight loss. These are collectively known as the "BRAVE" effects.[2]

The most discrete pathways of weight loss after RYGB are early satiety, calorie intake elimination, the possible increase in energy expenditure and the alteration in eating habits as patients postoperatively prefer foods which contain lower fat and less sugar than those they used to eat before the operation.[2] Dumping syndrome, which may appear as a complication after gastric bypass and less frequently after sleeve gastrectomy, may also be related to aversion or avoidance of food rich in fat and sugars.

The gut satiety hormones as well as the bile acids and the neuronal signals generated by the altered anatomy of the gut appear to play variable roles and are discussed elsewhere.

RYGB results in rapid weight loss in the first six months, followed by a plateau and eventually leads to 70–75% excess weight loss (EWL), which is equivalent to approximately 30% total body weight loss.

6.2.3. *Vertical Sleeve Gastrectomy*

The procedure begins with establishment of a pneumoperitoneum (Fig. 6.1(c)). The lesser sac is entered and the gastrocolic and gastrosplenic ligaments, as well as the lateral attachments of the stomach, are divided very close to and along the greater curve with the application of an energy device. The calibration of the remaining gastric lumen is done around a bougie or orogastric tube, the size of which varies between 32 and 44 French. The gastrectomy usually starts 2–10 cm proximal to the pylorus and extends to the fundus with the application of an endostapler. Some surgeons prefer to place a continuous suture over the staple line or use fibrin glue or omentum to secure it against haemorrhage or leak, whereas others use staple-line reinforcement materials at the time of firing the endostapler.

The specimen is extracted through one of the laparoscopic ports, which may require gentle widening. The operating time for the procedure is 45 min and the patients are discharged on the first postoperative day.

In the past, the procedure was chosen for high-risk patients as the first stage of a two-stage operation, the biliopancreatic diversion–duodenal switch (Fig. 6.1(d)). The complication rates are low including 1.2% for staple-line leakage, 1.6% for bleeding and 0.2% risk of mortality occurring within the first 30 postoperative days. The performance of the sleeve gastrectomy technique as a primary procedure and the use of staple-line reinforcements will likely further reduce the complication rate of the operation. The long-term compliance with nutrition is necessary, especially as long-term postoperative nutritional complications may occur due to the extensive gastric resection by decreasing the absorption of some vitamins and nutrients, such as vitamin B12 and iron.

Patients who underwent sleeve gastrectomy achieved 60–70% EWL, which is equivalent to approximately 25% total body weight loss, one year after surgery. The lack of long-term (>10 years) follow-up data remains the main concern regarding the evaluation of the effectiveness of the procedure.

The popularity of these two operations is decreasing due to the technical difficulties that characterise them as well as the higher risk of serious complications such as protein-calorie malnutrition, anaemia, bone mineral disease and vitamin deficiency. Nonetheless, these procedures result

Table 6.2.   Brief comparison of the current bariatric procedures.

Procedure	Gastric band	Gastric bypass	Sleeve gastrectomy
Duration	30–45 (minutes)	60–90 (minutes)	45–60 (minutes)
Hospital stay	Day case	2 days	1–2 days
Weight loss (first year)	20(%)	30(%)	25(%)
Mortality	0.01(%)	0.16(%)	0.02(%)
Advantages	• Reversible • Adjustable • Low early complication rate	• Rapid weight loss • Long term data • Suitable for sweet eaters	• No intestinal bypass • Satisfactory weight loss
Disadvantages	• Increased risk of malfunction or infection • Risk of band slippage or erosion — 10% reoperation • Regular follow-up	• Early serious complications (2%) • Long-term risk of bowel obstruction (1%)	• Early serious complications (1%) • No long-term data

in 80–90% EWL, which is equivalent to 40% total body weight loss, and provide the highest rates of resolution of the metabolic syndrome.

6.3. Clinical Outcome of Bariatric Surgery

The Swedish Obesity Subjects (SOS) study, conducted in Sweden, provides the largest follow-up outcomes after bariatric surgery (RYGB, VBG and gastric band).[3] Weight loss was maximal after 1 to 2 years; thus weight slowly increases until 8 to 10 years after surgery, when it stabilises. A decade following bariatric surgery the weight losses were 25% for gastric bypass and 14% for gastric banding.

In an updated systematic review and meta-analysis the five year weight loss outcomes after VSG seemed to be comparable with RYGB and appeared to be more effective than LAGB.

The prevalence of metabolic syndrome in obese patients is almost ten times higher compared to non-obese patients. The definition of the metabolic syndrome includes the coexistence of any three of the following five features: central obesity, high serum triglyceride levels, low serum high-density lipoprotein (HDL) levels, hypertension and elevated fasting blood glucose levels. According to Buchwald *et al.*, patients who undergo bariatric surgery achieved a 62% improvement of hypertension, 70% of hyperlipidaemia and 86% resolution of diabetes mellitus.[4]

Bariatric surgery was found to have a positive impact on the deceleration of atherosclerotic disease. Adams *et al.* found that the cause-specific mortality in the surgical group of patients decreased by 56% for coronary artery disease.[5] Also, according to Christou *et al.*, the risk of cardiovascular disease after bariatric surgery decreased by 72%.[6] Furthermore, bariatric surgery was found to improve heart systolic and diastolic performance and reduce left ventricular hypertrophy.

Obstructive sleep apnoea (OSA) and asthma represent common comorbidities for morbidly obese patients. According to the results of a systematic review and meta-analysis, sleep apnoea improved in 85% and resolved in 83% after bariatric surgery.[4] Severely obese patients with asthma experience resolution or improvement after bariatric surgery as well.

The SOS study reported that bariatric surgery had beneficial effects on diabetes, cardiovascular risk factors and symptoms, progression of intima–media thickness, sleep apnoea, joint pain, and health-related quality of life, and was also related to a marked reduction in overall mortality. In particular, during a follow up period up to 16 years, there was a 70% survival advantage in the surgical group. Moreover, Adams *et al.*, concluded that patients who underwent gastric bypass demonstrated significant improvements in most aspects of health related quality of life at six years compared with nonsurgical obese groups.[7]

According to Christou *et al.*, surgical intervention for treatment of obesity also significantly decreased overall mortality and the development of new health-related conditions in morbidly obese patients.[6]

In this study, patients who had bariatric surgery needed 50% fewer hospitalisations and had significantly reduced hospitalisation rates for cardiovascular conditions, infections, and respiratory conditions. On average, the total direct health care cost for the control patients was 45% higher compared with patients who underwent bariatric surgery.

6.4. Impact of Bariatric Surgery on Type 2 Diabetes (T2D)

Obesity and type 2 diabetes (T2D) are closely related and represent significant public health issues worldwide, thus the term "diabesity" was created to emphasise the close association between the above problems. T2D prevalence is increasing globally in parallel with obesity, and as many as 23% of patients with morbid obesity have T2D, whereas approximately 50% of those diagnosed with T2D are obese. Uncontrolled diabetes can cause macrovascular and microvascular complications, including myocardial infarction, stroke, vision loss, neuropathy and renal failure.

Obesity and T2D are difficult to control by current medical treatments, including diet, drug therapy and behavioural modification. Bariatric surgery is the most effective treatment of morbid obesity and, depending on the type of operation, is also very effective in the resolution of diabetes. This effect occurs even before the start of weight loss. The mechanisms underlying this are currently under study.

Weight loss, achieved through reduction of energy intake and increased exercise, is the foundation of treatment for T2D. According to the Look AHEAD trial, sustained weight loss via lifestyle modification results in improvement of diabetic control, but this is difficult to achieve and maintain over time. Medications to reduce hyperglycaemia and cardiovascular risk play an important role, but only up to 10% of patients with T2D manage to improve long-term risk of complications. The SOS study showed that patients after bariatric surgery had greater mean weight loss, reduced incidence of T2D, and less mortality than obesity-matched control patients. Randomised clinical

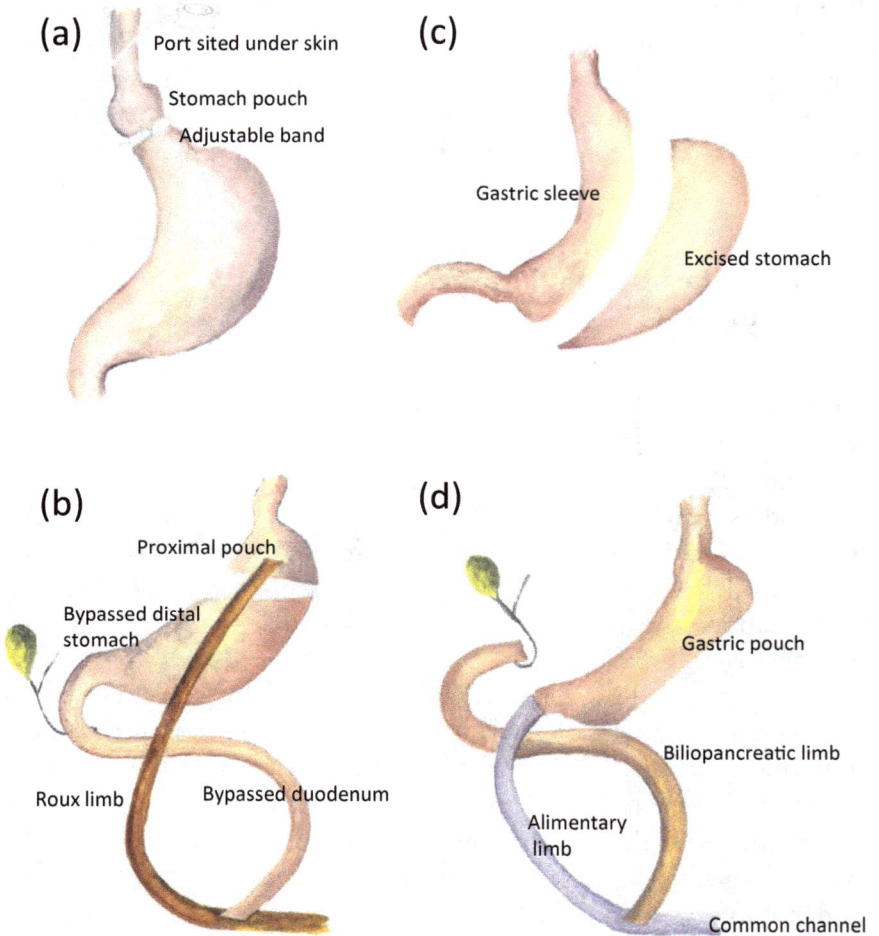

(a)
Port sited under skin
Stomach pouch
Adjustable band

(c)
Gastric sleeve
Excised stomach

(b)
Proximal pouch
Bypassed distal stomach
Roux limb
Bypassed duodenum

(d)
Gastric pouch
Biliopancreatic limb
Alimentary limb
Common channel

Figure 6.1.   (a) Adjustable gastric band; (b) Roux-en-Y gastric bypass; (c) Sleeve gastrectomy; (d) Biliopancreatic diversion with duodenal switch [Paintings by S. Zac-Varghese]

trials evaluating bariatric surgery as treatment for T2D have shown that LAGB, RYGB, VSG, and DS/BPD produced more weight loss and better glycaemic control than typical medical therapy.

Dixon *et al.* performed the first randomised clinical trial to compare the effectiveness of LAGB and conventional therapy in remission of T2D and reported significantly higher (73%) remission rates for the LAGB group compared with the conventional group (13%) after two years.[8] In another RCT study, Mingrone *et al.* concluded that after 2 years diabetes remission had occurred in 75% of patients undergoing gastric bypass and 95% undergoing BPD, whereas no remission of diabetes was reported for the patients who received medical therapy.[9] Moreover, according to the results of the recent STAMPEDE trial, after 3 years 38% of patients undergoing gastric bypass achieved glycaemic control with HbA1c < 6.0%, compared to 24 of patients undergoing laparoscopic sleeve gastrectomy and 5% of patients who received intensive medical therapy.[10] A recent meta-analysis of the current RCT data in available literature, published in BMJ, compared surgery with non-surgical treatment for obesity and concluded that at two years, bariatric surgery leads to greater weight loss and higher remission rates of T2D.[11] All studies related to the impact of bariatric surgery on the improvement or resolution of T2D demonstrated significant results in favour of the surgical intervention. Nonetheless, more studies are needed in order to evaluate the long-term (more than ten years) impact of bariatric surgery on T2D as well as on its microvascular complications.

6.5. Conclusions

- Laparoscopic adjustable gastric banding, Roux-en-Y gastric bypass and sleeve gastrectomy are the most popular procedures currently in use.
- Bariatric surgery is considered the most effective method of sustained weight loss as it has excellent long-term results and reduces comorbidities.
- Bariatric surgery results in improvement of T2D.

- More studies with long-term results are needed to demonstrate the effect of bariatric surgery on T2D and its microvascular complications.

References

1. O'Brien, P.E. (2010). Bariatric surgery: Mechanisms, indications and outcomes, *J. Gastroenterol. Hepatol.*, **25**(8), 1358–1365.
2. Ashrafian, H., Athanasiou, T., Li, J.V., Bueter, M., Ahmed, K., Nagpal, K., Holmes, E., Darzi, A. and Bloom, S.R. (2011). Diabetes resolution and hyperinsulinaemia after metabolic Roux-en-Y gastric bypass, *Obes. Rev.*, **12**(5), e257–272.
3. Sjöström, L., Narbro, K., Sjöström, D., Karason, K., Larsson, B., Wedel, H., Lystig, T., Sullivan, M., Bouchard, C., Carlsson, B., Bengtsson, C., Dahlgren, S., Gummesson, A., Jacobson, P., Karlsson, J., Lindroos, A.K., Lönroth, H., Näslund, I., Olbers, T., Stenlöf, K., Torgerson, J., Agren, G. and Carlsson, L.M.; Swedish Obese Subjects Study (2007). Effects of Bariatric Surgery on Mortality in Swedish Obese Subjects, *N. Engl. J. Med.*, **357**, 741–752.
4. Buchwald, H., Avidor, Y., Braunwald, E., Jensen, M.D., Pories, W., Fahrbach, K. and Schoelles, K. (2004). Bariatric surgery: A systematic review and meta-analysis, *JAMA*, **K292**(14), 1724–1737.
5. Adams, T.D., Gress, R.E., Smith, S.C., Halverson, R.C., Simper, S.C., Rosamond, W.D., Lamonte, M.J., Stroup, A.M. and Hunt, S.C. (2007). Long-term mortality after gastric bypass surgery, *N. Engl. J. Med.*, **357**(8), 753–761.
6. Christou, N.V., Sampalis, J.S., Liberman, M., Look, D., Auger, S., McLean, A.P. and MacLean, L.D. (2004). Surgery decreases long-term mortality, morbidity, and health care use in morbidly obese patients, *Ann. Surg.*, **240**, 416–424.
7. Kolotkin, R., Davidson, L.E., Crosby, R.D., Hunt S.C. and Adams, T.D. (2012). Six-year changes in health-related quality of life in gastric bypass patients versus obese comparison groups, *Surg. Obes. Relat. Dis.*, **8**(5), 625–633.
8. Dixon, J.B., O'Brien, P.E., Playfair, J., Chapman, L., Schachter, L.M., Skinner, S., Proietto, J., Bailey, M. and Anderson, M. (2008). Adjustable gastric banding and conventional therapy for type 2 diabetes: a randomized controlled trial, *JAMA*, **299**(3), 316–323.
9. Mingrone, G., Panunzi, S., De Gaetano, A., Guidone, C., Iaconelli, A., Leccesi, L., Nanni, G., Pomp, A., Castagneto, M., Ghirlanda, G. and Rubino, F. (2012). Bariatric surgery versus conventional medical therapy for type 2 diabetes, *N. Engl. J. Med.*, **366**, 1577–1585.
10. Schauer, P.R., Bhatt, D.L., Kirwan, J., Wolski, K., Brethauer, S.A., Navaneethan, S.D., Aminian, A., Pothier, C.E., Kim, E.S., Nissen, S.E. and Kashyap, S.R.; STAMPEDE Investigators (2014). Bariatric surgery versus

intensive medical therapy for diabetes — 3-year outcomes, *N. Engl. J. Med.*, **370**, 2002–2013.

11. Gloy, V., Briel, M., Bhatt, D.L., Kashyap, S.R., Schauer, P.R., Mingrone, G., Bucher, H.C. and Nordmann, A.J. (2013). Bariatric surgery versus non-surgical treatment for obesity: a systematic review and meta-analysis of randomised controlled trials, *BMJ*, **347**, f5934.

Chapter 7

GLP-1 in Bariatric Surgery and Diabetes: Underlying Molecular Mechanisms

N.B. Jørgensen and J.J. Holst

Department of Endocrinology, Hvidovre Hospital, Denmark and Panum Institute, University of Copenhagen, Denmark

7.1. Introduction

The best treatment for obesity as well as type 2 diabetes (T2D) is weight loss, but the chances of success through conventional methods, which are mainly lifestyle alterations, are limited. Dieting and exercise can produce weight losses of about 8–10% of body weight and, with the addition of anti-obesity drugs, a further weight loss of 2–8 kg may be obtainable. However, the problem with this approach is long-term maintenance of weight loss, as the patient will start to regain weight within less than a year when motivation fails and medical treatment is terminated. Over time, as many as 90% of patients will have returned to or exceeded the pre-intervention weight. As weight loss maintenance is important for producing lasting health benefits, it has been difficult to demonstrate reduction in obesity-associated morbidities or mortality in weight loss studies. This relative failure of lifestyle interventions has paved the way for more radical approaches. During the last 40 years, bariatric surgery, which treats obesity and comorbidities effectively through changes in energy intake and glucose metabolism, has gained popularity as a means of weight loss for morbidly obese individuals (BMI > 40). A number of different bariatric surgical procedures have been conceived, but those most frequently employed are laparoscopic adjustable gastric banding (LABG), vertical sleeve gastrectomy (VSG) and Roux-en-Y gastric bypass (RYGB).

LABG is a procedure whereby an adjustable silicon band is placed around the proximal stomach to create a small pouch. This mechanical restriction of the stomach results in a reduced effective stomach volume that is rapidly filled, causing wall distension when patients eat, thus inducing satiety, reduced energy intake and eventually weight loss.

The VSG procedure is a conversion of the gastric body into a narrow tube along the lesser curvature while the rest of the stomach is excised. The rationale here is the same as for the LABG, i.e. restriction of stomach volume.

RYGB on the other hand is a surgical remodelling of the gastrointestinal tract; a small pouch is created around the oesophagus, the small intestine is transected, typically 80–150 cm distally to the ligament of Treitz, the distal limb is anastomosed to the gastric pouch, while the proximal limb of the small intestine is anastomosed to a more distal part of the small intestine. The pouch was originally conceived as a restrictive element, but as it turns out, there is almost no retention of food here after a meal. The result is that orally ingested foods pass directly from the oesophagus to more distal parts of the small intestine.

Whilst the positive effect of LABG on T2D glucose metabolism relies on the magnitude of the postoperative weight loss, improved glucose tolerance is seen within days after RYGB surgery when patients have lost little weight. This is accompanied by dramatic increases in the postprandial secretion of glucagon-like peptide 1 (GLP-1) and other gut hormones. Consequently, much attention has been paid to gut hormones in general and incretin hormones in particular as potential contributors to these weight-loss-independent changes in glucose metabolism.

It is the aim of this chapter to review the disturbed incretin physiology in patients with T2D and to describe how this is influenced by bariatric surgery, with special focus on RYGB. Furthermore, the chapter provides an overview of key experimental approaches for evaluating incretin physiology and the challenges that remain in the field.

7.2. Review of the Field

The defects responsible for the loss of the incretin effect in T2D can occur at two levels: at the level of the gut, i.e. a reduced secretion of GIP and GLP-1, and at the level of the β cells, where the effect of incretin hormone stimulation may be attenuated or absent.

7.2.1. *Alterations in Incretin Secretion in T2D*

Glucose-dependent insulinotropic polypeptide (GIP) is released from entero-endocrine K cells in the proximal small intestine in response to luminal nutrients. Several studies have investigated GIP secretion in T2D, but results are ambiguous. In one large study in patients with normal glucose tolerance and T2D, Toft-Nielsen *et al.* found GIP secretion in response to a solid mixed breakfast meal to be modestly decreased compared to the responses of normal glucose-tolerant subjects, individually matched for gender, age and BMI.[1] However, a recent meta-analysis including 23 different studies and totalling a number of 363 patients found that neither peak GIP nor total GIP secretion in response to oral glucose load or a meal were decreased in T2D. Nevertheless, an increased HbA1c was significantly associated with a reduced GIP response. Obesity, on the other hand, was associated with increased GIP secretion.[2]

Entero-endocrine L cells responsible for GLP-1 secretion are unevenly distributed throughout the entire gastrointestinal epithelium, with high density in the ileum and the distal colon. However, there are indications that most of the meal-stimulated secretion actually derives from the proximal small intestine. Secretion is stimulated by luminal carbohydrates, fats, oligopeptides, amino acids and bile. When comparing the secretion of GLP-1 in patients with T2D, it is very important that the control group is well matched, especially with respect to BMI, as this has proven a very powerful predictor of the GLP-1 response: the higher the BMI, the lower the postprandial GLP-1 secretion. How BMI affects GLP-1 secretion is not fully elucidated, but recent reports suggest that hepatic steatosis plays an important role. In the previously mentioned study by Toft-Nielsen *et al.* where a solid breakfast meal was served, postprandial GLP-1 secretion was also measured, and here a rather pronounced reduction (~50%) in the late phase GLP-1 secretion (after 1 h) was found in T2D patients compared to normal glucose-tolerant controls. A similar impairment has not been identified in all studies, but many factors may be responsible for the variability. One possible explanation could be the nature of the meal. Because gastric emptying may be compromised in T2D as a result of hyperglycaemia, solid meals are probably retained for a longer time in the stomach than liquid meals/glucose solutions are. Since the magnitude of GLP-1 secretion is dependent on the rate of appearance of nutrients in the intestinal lumen, the nature of the oral stimulus (liquid/solid) could play a role and explain why some studies find decreased GLP-1 responses in patients with T2D and others do not. Indeed, in a meta-analysis of the GLP-1 response to oral stimulation in patients with T2D, GLP-1 secretion was found to be decreased in patients compared to controls only after solid meals and not after liquid meals or glucose suspensions. Other confounding factors include BMI, with many studies confirming an inverse relationship. Differences in insulin sensitivity may also play a role, as well as differences in gastric emptying rates (independent of the nature of the meal). The rate of gastric emptying is an extremely important determinant for GLP-1 secretion. Finally, presence or absence (wash-out) of anti-diabetic treatment may be important, particularly for metformin, which upregulates GLP-1 secretion.

In conclusion, postprandial secretion of GLP-1 is often reduced in T2D, and may of course contribute when present, but it is also clear that defects responsible for the diminished incretin effect may be found at the level of the β cells.

7.2.2. *Alterations in Incretin Sensitivity in T2D*

It has been known for decades now that GIP, even in supraphysiologi-cal doses, is not or only weakly insulinotropic during conditions of hyperglycaemia in patients with T2D. In contrast, pharmacological doses of GLP-1 have the potential to near-normalise insulin secretion in the same patients under the same circumstances. When considering that the intracellular signaling machinery, at least for a large part, is the same regardless of whether the extracellular stimulus is GIP or GLP-1, and considering that in T2D there is little or no GIP secre-tory defect, it follows that the GIP dysfunction might be related to the GIP receptor. It has been debated whether or not a GIP receptor defect contributes to the development of T2D and/or whether hyperglycaemia may influence its function. In one study, first-degree relatives of patients with T2D were found to have a reduced response to exogenous GIP infusion compared to healthy controls without a family history of T2D.[3] However, a later study performed under eug-lycaemic conditions could not detect differences in the insulinotropic effects of GIP in first degree relatives and controls.[4] A loss of function mutation of the human GIP receptor only had a marginal effect on glucose tolerance. Thus GIP receptor dysfunction might be a result of hyperglycaemia, which is supported by the finding that patients with diabetes on the basis of chronic pancreatitis (who probably only have hyperglycaemia in common with patients with T2D) have a reduced insulin secretory response to GIP infusion during a hypergly-caemic clamp compared to normal glucose-tolerant patients with chronic pancreatitis (a finding analogous to the differences found between patients with T2D and normal glucose-tolerant controls). *In vitro* studies in rodents and human islets of Langerhans have shown down-regulation of the GIP receptor when incubated in mod-erately high (>10 mmol/L) glucose concentrations for more than 24 h. Further support for hyperglycaemia as a cause for the loss of GIP effect on β cells comes from the observation that intensive insu-lin treatment in patients with T2D to lower glucose concentrations to near normal levels for four weeks partly restored the insulin response to GIP. Whilst β cell response to GIP is lost, a marked insulinotropic effect of GLP-1 is preserved in T2D. Thus, infusion of GLP-1 to slightly supraphysiological concentrations was capable of near-normalising the insulin secretory response to mildly elevated plasma glucose concentrations in patients with relatively mild T2D. Likewise, in a graded glucose infusion protocol, intravenous GLP-1 was able to normalise the integrated glucose response in patients with T2D compared to healthy controls, and to increase the insulin secretion of β cells in response to increments in plasma glucose concentrations (known as β cell glucose sensitivity) to equal to that of normal glucose-tolerant controls receiving saline infusion.[5] The preserved effect of GLP-1 in T2D is the rationale for the use of incretin based therapies, which include dipeptidyl peptidase-IV (DPP-IV) inhibitors and GLP-1 analogues. However, despite the pronounced stimulatory action of GLP-1 on insulin secretion in T2D, the dose–response relationship between GLP-1 and insulin secretion is impaired in patients when compared to healthy controls. Similar to what was found for the GIP receptor, there is evidence to suggest that the GLP-1 receptor is down regulated by "glucose toxicity", i.e. prolonged hyperglycaemia. This, in turn, would lead to GLP-1 resistance and a diminished effect on β cells. Hyperglycaemia is one metabolic feature of T2D; another is elevation of non-esterified fatty acids (NEFA). Chronically elevated NEFA concentrations are associated with reduced β cell function and one study reported that GLP-1 signaling was directly affected under such conditions, at least *in vitro*, where palmitate treatment led to down-regulation of GLP-1 receptor mRNA in insulinoma cells and β cells of isolated mouse islets, and reduced insulin secretion upon GLP-1 stimulation. Under the same circumstances, GIP receptor mRNA was not significantly suppressed.

The loss of incretin effect in patients with T2D thus represents a combination of the loss of responsiveness to GIP and a reduced sensitivity to GLP-1 of the pancreatic β cells. However, when considering impairment of incretin hormone effects on insulin secretion it is important to take β cell mass into account. β cell mass may be reduced in T2D (though this remains a controversial issue — for instance the remission of diabetes after gastric bypass is not due to proliferation of β cells, but to better performance of existing cells), and that in itself may cause the insulinotropic response of incretin hormone stimulation to be decreased compared to controls with normal glucose tolerance (and normal β cell mass). However, in obese normal glucose-tolerant subjects, who are generally considered to have an increased β cell mass and who have a many-fold increased risk of developing T2D, the incretin effect is impaired, demonstrating that disturbances in the incretin system may be present very early in the development of T2D.

As mentioned in Section 7.1, bariatric surgery has profound effects on glucose metabolism, but the magnitude of these effects depends on the type of surgery employed. Generally speaking, procedures that induce greater weight losses, like RYGB, are more likely to result in prolonged remission of T2D, compared to procedures with less dramatic effects on body weight, such as LABG and VSG. In a large meta-analysis including more than 600 studies and more than 100,000 patients, 80.3% of patients undergoing RYGB experienced remission of T2D, whereas this was only the case in 56.7% of patients undergoing LABG (numbers depend heavily on the definition of the term "remission"). The corresponding weight losses were 60% and 44% of excess body weight respectively. In a randomised clinically controlled study where the efficacy of RYGB or VSG in combination with medical therapy in inducing weight loss and lowering glucose levels were compared to medical therapy alone, patients treated with RYGB lost more weight and needed less additional medications to reach the target HbA1c level of 6.0% than patients treated with VSG.[6]

One very interesting feature of RYGB is the swiftness with which the effects on glucose metabolism occur. The day after the operation, and before any major weight loss, fasting glucose concentrations are greatly reduced, and patients can discard their anti-diabetic medication. Such rapid improvements in glycaemia are not seen after LABG, indicating that weight-loss-independent mechanisms contribute to diabetes remission after RYGB. Consequently, to better understand the changes taking place in glucose metabolism after surgery, RYGB-operated patients have been subject to intense physiological studies.

Some of the earliest studies addressed changes in fasting insulin and glucose concentrations a couple of weeks after RYGB.

The product of these two values, HOMA-IR (homeostatic measurement assessment — insulin resistance), provides a measure of insulin resistance (i.e. the inverse of insulin sensitivity), particularly at the level of the liver, and these studies, therefore, indicated that insulin sensitivity increases early after RYGB, irrespective of preoperative glucose tolerance status. Further studies, using intravenous glucose tolerance tests in both patients with T2D and normal glucose tolerance (NGT), confirmed that insulin sensitivity is improved early after surgery. Further studies employing the more laborious but also more accurate euglycaemic hyperinsulinaemic clamp in combination with glucose tracer infusion for the measurement of insulin sensitivity confirmed that early after RYGB, hepatic insulin sensitivity increased, whereas muscle insulin sensitivity did not increase until one to three months after the operation. There are several studies suggesting that the acute changes in hepatic insulin sensitivity are due to the caloric restriction present immediately after surgery, whereas peripheral insulin sensitivity improves as patients lose weight. Data on insulin sensitivity early after LABG are not as abundant, but in general, insulin sensitivity improves with weight loss, perhaps reflecting that early caloric restriction is not as intense after LABG as after RYGB.

Given the fact that gastrointestinal continuity is changed after RYGB and that orally ingested foods bypass the major part of the stomach, the duodenum and the first part of the small intestine, much interest has been focussed on gastrointestinal factors and not least on incretin hormones. Early on, experiments in rodents suggested that exclusion of the foregut could lead to improvements in glucose metabolism, which in turn led to the so-called proximal gut hypothesis, which claimed that bypass of the proximal gut caused a decreased secretion of an "anti-incretin". This "anti-incretin" has never been identified, and currently evidence points towards an increased stimulation of the distal gut as the key mediator of the improvements in glucose metabolism.

After RYGB, β cell function is largely unchanged in NGT and T2D patients as determined after an intravenous glucose stimulation, but when oral glucose is used as a stimulus instead, β cell function is greatly improved. This effect is most pronounced in patients with

T2D, but if concurrent improvements in insulin sensitivity are taken into account, β cell function is also improved in non-diabetic RYGB operated subjects. After oral ingestion of a meal, food passes directly into the small intestine without retention in the gastric pouch. Thus, luminal concentrations of nutrients are greatly increased in the more distal parts of the small intestine, where L cells are located in high numbers, and this stimulates the secretion of gut-hormones such as peptide YY (PYY) and GLP-1. Early on, Laferrere *et al.* explored the effect of RYGB on the incretin effect, which was normalised in patients with T2D after RYGB when compared to obese glucose tolerant controls.[7] Later studies showed that diabetic patients undergoing diet-induced weight loss similar to a group of RYGB operated patients did not experience this improvement in the incretin effect.[8] In these studies, the improved incretin effect was associated with increased GLP-1 and GIP secretion. However, while a dramatically (up to 20-fold) increased GLP-1 secretion in response to oral stimulation has been demonstrated in a large number of studies, GIP secretion varies, and has been found to be both decreased, increased and unchanged after RYGB. Hypersecretion of GLP-1 is not seen after caloric restriction or LABG, but some studies indicate that VSG-operated patients have a similar response to meals. Thus, after RYGB, in addition to improved insulin sensitivity, the incretin effect is normalised and β cell function improved following oral stimulation.

The obvious mechanism responsible would be the increased GLP-1 secretion, and this has been investigated in a few studies, where meal stimulation has been carried out in the absence and presence of exendin-9 (Ex9), a GLP-1 receptor antagonist. These studies show, unequivocally, that GLP-1 is the major driver of the improved β cell function after RYGB. In fact, β cell function can be brought back to preoperative levels in patients with preoperative T2D by blocking the GLP-1 receptor.[9]

As previously pointed out, in T2D the incretin defect is mainly at the level of the β cells, where β cell sensitivity to GLP-1 and especially GIP is reduced, perhaps due to metabolic effects (hyperglycaemia, hyperlipidaemia). As both glucose concentrations and triglyceride concentrations decrease in patients with T2D after RYGB, β cell sensitivity to GLP-1 and GIP may be increased. The operation *per se* does not have the potential to change the β cell sensitivity to incretin hormones substantially. This has been investigated in non-diabetic patients, who were subjected to a hyperglycaemic clamp with infusion of saline, GIP and GLP-1 on separate study days, and the incretin hormones were just as insulinotropic before the operation as they were after. Whether this is true in patients with T2D, who experience large metabolic changes following RYGB, remains to be shown.

Apart from the effects directly on α and β cells, GLP-1 is also involved in the regulation of hunger and satiety. GLP-1 infusion leads to reduced *ad libitum* energy intake in healthy subjects, and patients with T2D treated with GLP-1 analogues lose weight during treatment, which contributes to the improved glucose regulation. Because postprandial GLP-1 secretion is dramatically increased after RYGB, energy intake could be decreased as a consequence. Furthermore, there are findings to support a role for GLP-1 in determining weight loss after surgery. For instance, patients with a poor weight-loss response have a reduced GLP-1 secretion in response to meals compared to patients with a good weight-loss response. On the other hand, these findings could be simply due to the differences in body weight in the two groups. Nevertheless, the idea of gut hormones contributing to weight loss after RYGB by down-regulating energy intake is a compelling one. GLP-1 is not the only gut hormone hypersecreted after the operation; a number of other potent anorexigenic gut hormones, including PYY, cholecystokinin (CCK), oxyntomodulin and neurotensin, are also secreted in exaggerated amounts after a meal. From studies in animals and humans it is well known that these gut hormones have additive and perhaps even synergistic effects on food intake, being more anorexigenic when infused together than when given alone. Weight loss is crucial for the increase in insulin sensitivity after surgery and it is very important in maintaining diabetes remission. Thus, GLP-1 and other gut hormones may improve glucose tolerance after RYGB not just by influencing β cells directly to produce more insulin, but also by reducing energy intake and promoting weight loss.

7.3. Key Experimental Approaches

The incretin effect designates the amplification of insulin secretion after an oral glucose challenge as opposed to an intravenous glucose infusion to provide identical plasma glucose concentrations, and this definition also provides an idea as to how the incretin effect is studied. Two experimental days are needed to conduct the two procedures: an oral glucose tolerance test (OGTT) and an isoglycaemic intravenous glucose infusion (IIGI) to match the plasma glucose values obtained on the day of the OGTT.

7.3.1. *Day 1 — OGTT*

1. Subject undergoes an overnight fast.
2. Baseline blood samples are drawn at –20 min, –10 min and 0 min.
3. Subject consumes a standardised glucose suspension (typically containing 75 g of glucose) over 5 min.
4. Frequent blood sampling is necessary, especially during the first hour, where changes in plasma glucose concentrations occur at a rapid rate.

7.3.2. *Day 2 — IIGI*

1. Subject undergoes an overnight fast.
2. Baseline blood samples are drawn at –20 min, –10 min and 0 min.
3. 20% glucose solution is infused intravenously to match glucose concentrations measured on day 1. This is done by continuously adjusting the infusion rate of glucose (usually around 20–25 g in total need to be infused).
4. Blood is sampled at the same time points as during the OGTT.
5. To evaluate the incretin effect, insulin concentrations need to be determined.

Often, the intention is to describe the effect of an intervention on the incretin effect, and whether this intervention affects hepatic insulin clearance. C-peptide concentrations are a better measure of β cell insulin secretion. Measurements of total GLP-1 and GIP concentrations to determine the level of incretin hormone secretion during the OGTT can be added to characterise the effects of an intervention further.

The calculation of the incretin effect relies on incremental areas of insulin/C-peptide; thus, a couple of important points must be taken into account when planning experiments. Firstly, establishing reliable baseline values is very important and requires three baseline samples. Secondly, the time of observation after the OGTT, must be long enough to allow insulin/C-peptide concentrations to return to baseline values, which means that experiments must last at least 180 min and preferably 240 min, especially if diabetic subjects are studied.

7.3.3. *The Hyperglycaemic Clamp*

The hyperglycaemic clamp with incretin hormone infusions is a method for studying β cell sensitivity to incretin hormones. The principle is simple in theory: plasma glucose is elevated to levels that stimulate insulin secretion by a continuous glucose infusion and kept constant for a one-hour to two-hour period. Before glucose infusion starts, baseline values are determined, and during glucose infusion blood is sampled frequently to adjust the glucose infusion and for measurement of insulin and C-peptide concentrations. This experimental procedure yields two different measures of β cell function:

(1) The first phase response or the acute insulin response (AIR) is considered a measure of the number of insulin-containing granules available for immediate release in response to increments in plasma glucose concentrations. This is impaired or absent in patients with diabetes.

(2) The second phase response represents a measure of complex intracellular processes in the β cells, encompassing insulin synthesis, packaging of insulin in vesicles, transport of vesicles to the plasma membrane and fusion of vesicles with the plasma membrane in response to elevated plasma glucose concentrations; this is impaired to a varying degree in T2D.

The above represents the basic hyperglycaemic clamp. For testing β cell sensitivity to incretin hormones, this needs to be repeated on separate days with infusion of placebo, GLP-1 and/or GIP. The insulinotropic effects of incretin hormones on the first-phase and second-phase insulin responses can then be quantified by comparing the placebo day with hormone days.

While the basic principle is simple, there are a couple of important points that need consideration when planning experiments using the hyperglycaemic clamp. Often the effect of an intervention on β cell function in patients with T2D is studied, but if this intervention has profound effects on glucose metabolism, as seen after RYGB, then the baseline glucose concentration from where hyperglycaemia is induced varies greatly across the intervention. If a fixed hyperglycaemic glucose concentration is chosen, then the increment in plasma glucose concentrations can differ quite dramatically before and after the intervention, which translates into differing glucose stimulation of the β cells. This can be circumvented through an approach where hyperglycaemia is not fixed at a given value, but instead a fixed elevation of glucose concentrations is used. Pre- and post-intervention studies will then have the same increment in plasma glucose concentrations, but will be conducted at different absolute glucose concentrations, which may be a problem. A third way is to normalise baseline glucose concentrations using a fast-acting insulin analogue before starting the clamp at all study points. Furthermore, a primed incretin hormone infusion is warranted, if the effect of GLP-1 and/or GIP on the first phase response is investigated.

7.3.4. *Graded Glucose Infusion*

Another method for studying β cell sensitivity to incretin hormones is the graded glucose infusion. After establishing baseline values, a stepwise increment in plasma glucose concentration is obtained through a graded intravenous glucose infusion, each step lasting 30 to 40 minutes. Blood samples for insulin, C-peptide and glucose concentrations are drawn. Thus a dose–response relationship can be established and because C-peptide measurements are used for calculating pre-hepatic insulin secretion through deconvolution, it is possible to correlate glucose concentrations with β cell insulin secretion, allowing for determination of a β cell glucose dose–response relationship. The graded glucose infusion test can then be carried out on different days with infusions of placebo, GLP-1, or GIP.

7.3.5. *Meal Tests*

The physiological role of incretins may be studied in meal tests, where the endogenous incretin hormone secretion is stimulated. When the meal test is carried out in the presence and absence of incretin hormone receptor antagonists, such as the GLP-1 receptor antagonist Ex9, the changes in glucose, insulin and C-peptide concentrations, the effects of endogenous GLP-1 become evident, compared to a normal meal test. Suitable GIP receptor antagonists for human use are not yet available.

Here the focus has been on *in vivo* experiments, but incretin hormone effects have also been extensively studied in *in vitro* models (Chapter 3).

7.4. Key Challenges/Gaps in the Field

There is little doubt that the loss of the incretin effect in diabetes contributes importantly to the impaired insulin secretion, particularly viewed in the context of insulin resistance. But, as discussed above, it is not a primary event in the pathogenesis, but rather develops — although very early — in the course of the disease. Based on the early studies revealing decreased secretion of GLP-1 and loss of effect of GIP, combined with the ability of GLP-1 infusions to normalise insulin secretion and provide normoglycaemia, it was felt that GLP-1 therapy might be viewed as a substitution therapy, restoring the lost incretin effect. This view should not be maintained, since a therapy relying on GLP-1 agonism alone is unlikely to represent a lasting solution for many patients. The original enthusiasm regarding the β-cell-proliferating effects of GLP-1 has been replaced by recognition that GLP-1 may protect β cells, but cannot make adult β cells in humans (and experimental animals) proliferate. A GLP-1-based therapy of diabetes should recognise this: the basic (probably genetic) β cell failure cannot be addressed by incretins but requires other approaches, for instance combinations with basal insulin or maybe Na^+ glucose co-transporter 2 (SGLT-2) inhibitors. Such combinations have proven exceedingly effective, with often up to 80% of the patients reaching an HbA1c target of less than 7%, in combination with weight loss and lesser hypoglycaemia.

It remains a riddle why GIP loses its effect in T2D, while GLP-1 remains effective. Further studies of the intracellular events elicited in β cells by the two hormones should be carried out to elucidate this, since the difference is likely to be related to the fundamental issue of the failure of glucose to stimulate insulin secretion in the diabetic β cell. Insight into these mechanisms might lead to new essential pharmacological approaches.

The weight loss caused by GLP-1 alone is moderate (around 5–10 % of initial body weight), and although it has been possible to use larger doses than originally anticipated (with correspondingly greater efficacy), it seems difficult to employ higher doses still because of the side effects. The levels of (endogenous) GLP-1 observed in peripheral plasma after RYGB correspond to very high hormone levels in the splanchnic bed (possibly interacting with sensory afferent neurons signalling to the brain stem and hypothalamus), which could not be reproduced by injection/infusion without severe side effects. A better way to utilise the incretin systems would therefore apparently be to stimulate the endogenous secretion, as this occurs after RYGB, and many research groups are currently trying to understand how this could be done (Chapter 2).

RYGB is by far the best studied bariatric surgery procedure due to the fact that it has been the most widely used form of bariatric surgery for a number of years. As a direct consequence, many aspects of RYGB physiology are now established. We know that the incretin effect is increased and that β cell function is improved in patients with T2D after RYGB, due mainly to an increased GLP-1 secretion in relation to meals.

This is not an effect of weight loss, but rather of the operation itself, which leads to an increased presentation of nutrients to the distal part of the small intestine. This was clearly illustrated in a case study where a patient was studied five weeks after RYGB with a meal test on two consecutive days. On one day he was fed orally, on the other via a gastrostomy catheter introduced into the disconnected stomach, i.e. via the "normal" route. Only on the day where the stomach/upper small intestine was bypassed, did he have exaggerated GLP-1 secretion (and on that day he was glucose tolerant, while diabetic on the other).[10]

It remains to be determined if patients with T2D have an increased β cell sensitivity to GLP-1 and GIP after the operation. Also, the effect of the operation on food intake and body weight is probably due to the hypersecretion of a combination of gut hormones, including PYY and perhaps oxyntomodulin as discussed above, but how GLP-1 and other gut hormones contribute to reduce the post-surgery energy intake and cause weight loss is not yet completely understood. In this context, description of the gut–brain interaction after RYGB is of great interest. Therapies based on combinations of such hormones might be effective, not only in terms of weight loss, but also in terms of diabetes therapy since the weight loss alone would bring about remission of the disease in a high number of patients.

Patients who have received a VSG do not have quite as high a rate of diabetes remission after surgery as patients with RYGB. However, many of the metabolic changes found after RYGB appear to be present in VSG-operated patients also. Thus, GLP-1 secretion is similarly increased and β cell function probably improved, most likely because of a similarly accelerated nutrient entry into the small intestine. The procedure has not been characterised to the same extent, because it has only gained popularity for treating obesity within recent years.

7.5. Conclusions

- The loss of incretin effect is not the cause of T2D, but a very early feature of the disease.
- T2D patients practically lose β cell responsivity to GIP, whereas GLP-1 remains insulinotrophic. The retained effect of GLP-1 in T2D is the rationale for the use of incretin-based therapies.

- The incretin deficiency is partly due to the metabolic phenotype of T2D, with elevated plasma glucose and lipid concentrations.
- Early after RYGB, GLP-1 secretion is greatly exaggerated, and this results in an improved (normalised) incretin effect and in improved β cell function in patients with T2D upon oral glucose stimulation.
- The hypersecretion of GLP-1 and other anorexigenic gut hormones (such as PYY and oxyntomodulin) most likely reduces caloric intake and leads to weight loss and improved insulin sensitivity after RYGB.
- RYGB may serve as a model for the design of future diabetes medications.

References

1. Toft-Nielsen, M.B., Damholt, M.B., Madsbad, S., Hilsted, L.M., Hughes, T.E., Michelsen, B.K. and Holst, J.J. (2001). Determinants of the impaired secretion of glucagon-like peptide-1 in type 2 diabetic patients, *J. Clin. Endocrinol. Metab.*, **86**(8), 3717–3723.
2. Calanna, S., Christensen, M., Holst, J.J., Laferrère, B., Gluud, L.L., Vilsbøll, T. and Knop, F.K. (2013). Secretion of glucagon-like peptide-1 in patients with type 2 diabetes mellitus: Systematic review and meta-analyses of clinical studies, *Diabetologia*, **56**(5), 965–972.
3. Meier, J., Holst, J. and Deacon, C. (2001). Reduced insulinotropic effect of gastric inhibitory polypeptide in first-degree relatives of patients with type 2 diabetes, *Diabetes*, **50**(11), 2497–2504.
4. Meier, J.J., Nauck, M.A., Siepmann, N., Greulich, M., Holst, J.J., Deacon, C.F., Schmidt, W.E. and Gallwitz, B. (2003). Similar insulin secretory response to a gastric inhibitory polypeptide bolus injection at euglycemia in first-degree relatives of patients with type 2 diabetes and control subjects, *Metabolism*, **52**(12), 1579–1585.
5. Kjems, L.L., Holst, J.J., Vølund, A. and Madsbad, S. (2003). The influence of GLP-1 on glucose-stimulated insulin secretion: effects on beta-cell sensitivity in type 2 and nondiabetic subjects, *Diabetes*, **44**(10), 380–386.
6. Schauer, P.R., Bhatt, D.L. and Kashyap, S.R. (2014). Bariatric surgery versus intensive medical therapy for diabetes--3-year outcomes, *N. Engl. J. Med.*, **370**(21), 2002–2013.
7. Laferrère, B., Heshka, S., Wang, K., Khan, Y., McGinty, J., Teixeira, J., Hart, A.B. and Olivan, B. (2007). Incretin levels and effect are markedly enhanced 1 month after Roux-en-Y gastric bypass surgery in obese patients with type 2 diabetes, *Diabetes Care*, **30**(7), 1709–1716.

8. Laferrère, B., Teixeira, J., McGinty, J., Tran, H., Egger, J.R., Colarusso, A., Kovack, B., Bawa, B., Koshy, N., Lee, H., Yapp, K. and Olivan, B. (2008). Effect of weight loss by gastric bypass surgery versus hypocaloric diet on glucose and incretin levels in patients with type 2 diabetes, *J. Clin. Endocrinol. Metab.*, **93**(7), 2479–2485.

9. Jørgensen, N.B., Dirksen, C., Bojsen-Møller, K.N., Jacobsen, S.H., Worm, D., Hansen, D.L., Kristiansen, V.B., Naver, L., Madsbad, S. and Holst, J.J. (2013). Exaggerated glucagon-like peptide 1 response is important for improved β-cell function and glucose tolerance after Roux-en-Y gastric bypass in patients with type 2 diabetes, *Diabetes*, **62**(9), 3044–3052.

10. Dirksen, C., Hansen, D.L., Madsbad, S., Hvolris, L.E., Naver, L.S., Holst, J.J., Worm, D. (2010). Postprandial diabetic glucose tolerance is normalized by gastric bypass feeding as opposed to gastric feeding and is associated with exaggerated GLP-1 secretion: a case report, *Diabetes Care*, **33**(2), 375–377.

Chapter 8

GLP-1-Based Therapies:
What are the Safety Implications?

A. Mondragon, A. Bertling, R. Gomes-Faria, G.A. Rutter
and G. da Silva Xavier

Department of Cell Biology, Imperial College London

8.1. Review of the Field

The incretin glucagon-like peptide 1 (GLP-1), secreted after meal ingestion, promotes the secretion of insulin and somatostatin by pancreatic β and δ cells, respectively (see Chapter 2). GLP-1 also decreases glucagon production from α cells (Chapter 4), as well as appetite and gastric emptying. Several studies have shown that GLP-1 administration exerted beneficial effects on other tissue systems, including the cardiovascular and nervous systems. These positive effects, as well as a suggested action on β cell proliferation and an absence of adverse effects such as weight gain and hypoglycaemic episodes, make GLP-1 an ideal candidate as a drug to treat type 2 diabetes (T2D).

The GLP-1 receptor (GLP-1R) agonist and dipeptidyl peptidase-IV (DPP-IV) inhibitor class of anti-diabetes drugs are relatively new additions to the list of anti-diabetes treatments. Although an efficient drug class for the treatment of T2D, recent data indicate that long-term administration of the GLP-1R agonists and DPP-IV inhibitors may be linked to an increased risk of pancreatitis and pancreatic cancer,[1-3] fuelling a debate as to the safety of these drugs. The risk of pancreatic cancer conferred by the usage of these anti-diabetic drugs is difficult to assess, as patients with a history of pancreatitis and diabetes are in any case at increased risk of developing pancreatic cancer.[4,5] The relative risk of pancreatic cancer in obese individuals has also been shown to be similar to the risks observed in diabetic individuals.

8.1.1. *GLP-1R Agonists and DPP-IV Inhibitors Linked to Pancreatitis and Pancreatic Cancer*

Three commonly used agents are exenatide/exendin-4 (Ex4) and liraglutide, which are GLP-1R agonists, and sitagliptin, a DPP-IV inhibitor. Most of the literature covering pancreatitis and pancreatic cancer risks involve the use of these three agents. Ex4, approved for the treatment of T2D in 2005, is a component of Gila monster venom. It is part of a complex mixture including exendin-3 that stimulates pancreatic enzyme release. It has been shown in a rat model of T2D that GLP-1 receptors are expressed in the exocrine pancreas, and prolonged exposure to sitagliptin increases pancreatic ductal replication, acinar to ductal metaplasia — both well-established characteristics of chronic pancreatitis in humans and acute pancreatitis. Low-grade pancreatitis has also been observed in rats treated with Ex4 for 75 days. These results raised concerns, as chronic pancreatitis has been shown to increase the risk of pancreatic cancer.[6]

Liraglutide, a once-daily alternative to Ex4, was approved for the treatment of T2D by the U.S. Food and Drug Administration (FDA) in 2010. It is structurally similar to GLP-1 and has a half-life of 11–15 hours. Liraglutide binds avidly to albumin, making it more stable. In total, liraglutide's efficacy and safety have been investigated in more than 5000 patients through 20 clinical trials. In a number of these studies markers of β cell function were also analysed, leading to the indication of improved β cell function. A recent report suggested that liraglutide might be more effective for glycaemic control than Ex4 in some patients due to the development of inhibitory antibodies against Ex4 in these individuals. Furthermore, there are initial indications that liraglutide functions to decrease the elevated expression of endothelin-1 in diabetic patients, leading to molecular changes associated with improvement of T2D but also with atherosclerosis. Possible beneficial effects of liraglutide against the development of atherosclerotic vascular disease have also been found in a rodent model.

Sitagliptin is a DPP-IV inhibitor that was approved for use as a treatment for T2D in 2005. GLP-1 is inactivated by DPP-IV through enzymatic cleavage to generate GLP-1_{9-39}, and DPP-IV inhibition is known to raise intact GLP-1 concentrations in the plasma. GLP-1 represents a high-affinity substrate for DPP-IV, although DPP-IV also inactivates glucose-dependent insulinotropic polypeptide (GIP), pituitary adenylate cyclase and gastrin-releasing peptide, some of which also play a role in glucose homeostasis, as well as possibly other peptides. This action thus forms an important distinction between the actions of the GLP-1 analogues and the DPP-IV class of inhibitor, both in terms of clinical efficacy and possible side effects. Sitagliptin exhibits high potency towards DPP-IV with an IC_{50} of 18 nM. It is normally administered orally once or twice daily, with steady-state plasma levels of sitagliptin reached within three days of administration, with an elimination half time of 12–14 h. Doses of 50–200 mg administered once per day have been shown to lead to over 80% inhibition of DPP-IV activity over 24 h, resulting in two- to three-fold increase in intact GLP-1 in the postprandial state. Sitagliptin is weight neutral, does not increase the incidence of hypoglycaemic episodes, and rodent data indicate that it may achieve improved glycaemic control through improved β cell function, survival and proliferation. However, recent analysis of VigiBase, the World Health Organisation Adverse Drug Reactions database, indicated that DPP-IV inhibitors may exert adverse effects on the immune system, thereby leading to an increase in the incidence of upper respiratory tract infections.

8.1.2. *Timeline of Safety Concerns*

Drug safety testing is carried out in stages (Fig. 8.1). For diabetes drugs, the regulatory requirements give (primal) importance to demonstration of lowering of HbA1c levels with no increase in cardiovascular risk. In 2009, the FDA issued a warning to healthcare professionals about the possible increased risk of pancreatitis in T2D patients taking sitagliptin following 88 cases of acute pancreatitis related to sitagliptin use; pancreatitis was also associated with exenatide use. Thereafter, more cases of acute pancreatitis associated with several GLP-1-based therapies have been reported. Examination of the FDA's Adverse Event Reporting System (AERS) database in 2004–2009 showed a six-fold increased odds ratio of reported pancreatitis for sitagliptin and Ex4 in comparison with other therapies.[7] A more recent study based on event numbers for acute pancreatitis and patient exposure to GLP-1 receptor agonists and DPP-IV

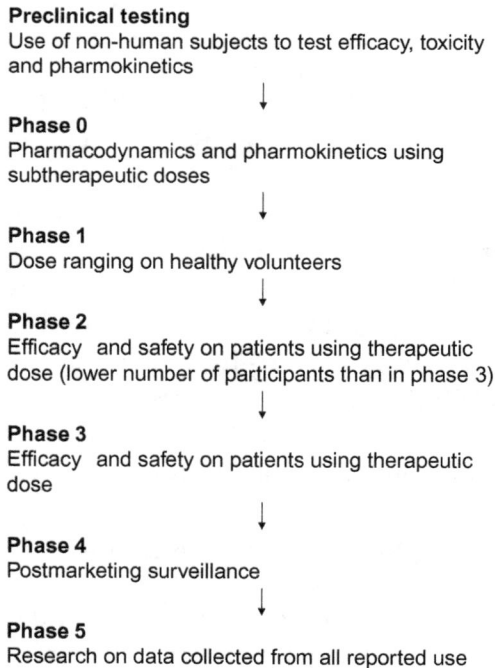

Preclinical testing
Use of non-human subjects to test efficacy, toxicity and pharmokinetics

↓

Phase 0
Pharmacodynamics and pharmokinetics using subtherapeutic doses

↓

Phase 1
Dose ranging on healthy volunteers

↓

Phase 2
Efficacy and safety on patients using therapeutic dose (lower number of participants than in phase 3)

↓

Phase 3
Efficacy and safety on patients using therapeutic dose

↓

Phase 4
Postmarketing surveillance

↓

Phase 5
Research on data collected from all reported use

Figure 8.1. Flowchart for drug safety testing.

inhibitors indicated a trend towards slightly elevated pancreatitis risk for patients on GLP-1 receptor agonists but not DPP-IV inhibitors. There is, nonetheless, a lack of information from human pancreata from patients on long-term treatment. The use of the AERS to assess drug safety is also arguably imperfect. Subsequently, it was reported that administration of GLP-1 receptor agonists or DPP-IV inhibitors was associated with increased serum amylase and lipase levels, which are indicative of pancreatitis. Ex4 was shown to accelerate the formation of neoplastic pancreatic intraepithelial (PanIN) lesions and to exacerbate chronic pancreatitis in mice. Studies linking liraglutide with increased or no incidence of pancreatitis were also subsequently published. In addition, the debate, previously chiefly confined to diabetes professionals, has now also reached patients, with implications for treatment adherence. The evidence for an association between GLP-1-based therapy and the development of pancreatitis is intensified by the fact that all of the developed agents that have been on the market long enough have now been linked to cases of pancreatitis. Moreover, a flurry of studies in rodents from Butler and colleagues,[7] demonstrating increased signs of pancreatitis, generated further cause for concern. Although much has been published on the potential risk of pancreatitis and pancreatic cancer from administration of GLP-1 mimetics, it must be borne in mind that some of the concerns may represent the effect of "over-repeating" for newly identified treatments. Indeed most meta-analyses failed to demonstrate significant increases in the risk of pancreatitis or pancreatic cancer.

Furthermore, there have equally been studies that demonstrate no effects on these parameters. For example, it has previously been shown that C57BL/6 mice do not develop pancreatitis following treatment with Ex4 for seven days; Zucker diabetic fatty rats administered exendatide or liraglutide for 13 weeks did not exhibit significant pancreatitis as assessed by qualitative histopathological analysis, but did exhibit small increases in P-amylase activity. A recent study by Ellenbroek and colleagues[8] demonstrated that mice administered liraglutide prior to the start of a six-week-long high-fat diet regimen remained normoglycaemic and exhibited decreased β cell mass, possibly due to improved insulin sensitivity.

In total, liraglutide's efficacy and safety have been investigated in more than 5000 patients through 20 clinical trials; in a number of these studies markers of β cell function were also analysed, leading to the indication of improved β cell function, amongst other potential beneficial effects. Data from non-human primates also indicate that liraglutide did not represent significant pancreatitis risk. The FDA and EMA (European Medicines Agency) expert panels have also recently (2014) ruled that available data do not confirm recent concerns over an increased risk for pancreatic side effects with GLP-1-based diabetes therapies.

A survey of the literature on incretin-based treatments reveals that there is potential for the use of these drugs for the treatment not only of diabetes and obesity, but also chronic inflammation, alcohol addiction and Alzheimer's disease. Of these, alcohol overuse may predispose to pancreatitis. There are several other agents in clinical trials that are also GLP-1 analogues. It is important, therefore, that we have information on the long-term effects of the use of incretin-based therapies.

8.2. Key Experimental Approaches and Challenges in the Field

Animal studies do not necessarily predict with certainty what will happen in humans during similar treatment protocols.[9] Nonetheless, given the poor prognosis for patients diagnosed with pancreatic cancer, and the lack of risk data from long term studies of patients on these treatments, there is a case argument for following long-term treatment with GLP-1R agonists in model systems. The discrepancies between the propensity for animal models to develop pancreatitis with or without GLP-1R agonist or DPP-IV inhibitor treatment in different studies may partly be explained by the disparities in the model systems used. In humans, obesity is associated with increased risk of T2D and pancreatitis/pancreatic cancer. Thus, it is possible that the pancreatitis risk seen in patients on GLP-1R agonists or DPP-IV inhibitor treatment may be mediated by both these factors — i.e. that obesity and drug treatment together may be the trigger. The model

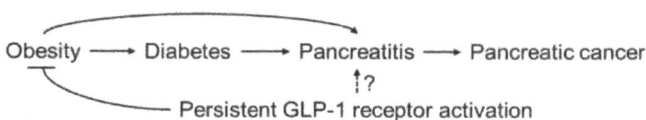

Figure 8.2. Does GLP-1 receptor activation lead to pancreatitis and pancreatic cancer? There is evidence linking obesity, diabetes, pancreatitis and pancreatic cancer. Recent data suggest that persistent GLP-1 receptor activation may lead to pancreatitis and pancreatic cancer but the mechanisms that lead to this are unclear.

systems and test treatment protocol should reflect these parameters. The basic question is illustrated in Fig. 8.2.

8.2.1. *Key Experimental Approaches*

We have addressed some of the above issues, particularly with regard to the effect of incretins in model (rodent) systems in a recent study.[10] Thus, we assessed the pancreatitis risk in mice administered one of liraglutide, Ex4 or sitagliptin by using a model of high-fat-induced hyperglycaemia, which reflects key elements of T2D in humans. Our experimental scheme is illustrated in Fig. 8.3. Thus, the drugs were administered to mice that already exhibited glucose dyshomeostasis. We used drug doses and administration routes with previously demonstrated efficacy for our model system, and a time period for treatment that has previously been reported to be sufficient to lead to pancreatitis, albeit in a different model system. There is much debate in the literature regarding how best to assess pancreatitis in rodents, so we incorporated all the suggested methods — histopathological assessment, immunohistochemistry for markers of pancreatitis, and plasma amylase and lipase measurements — in our workflow. We found that the drugs had different effects on pancreatitis risk in our model system and that the three methods used to assess pancreatitis risk gave widely varying readouts, which may be indicative of the relative sensitivities of the methods.

Histopathology is a qualitative method of analysis and requires access to experienced personnel with proficiency in looking at tissues from specific model systems. Whilst this is a valuable assessment tool,

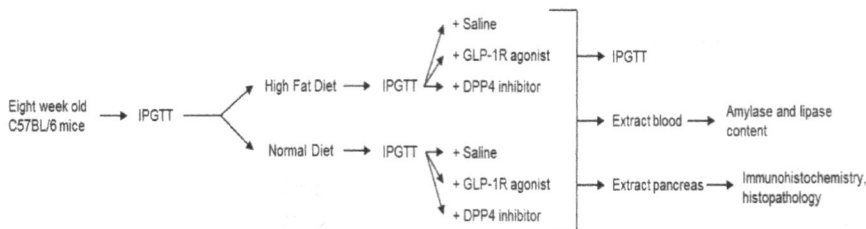

Figure 8.3. Experimental scheme. Mouse weights were recorded weekly through-out the experimental period. Mice were assessed for glycaemic control by intraperi-toneal glucose tolerance test (IPGTT) prior to the start of an eight-week diet regime, whereby mice were either administered normal chow diet or high-fat diet (60% fat). This induced glucose intolerance in the mice on high-fat diet, which was verified by IPGTT. The mice were then kept on the diet regime whilst being exposed to daily intraperitoneal injections of saline or GLP-1R agonist or DPP-IV inhibitor at the start of the dark cycle, for 75 days. At the end of the treatment period, mice were subjected to IPGTT to assess glucose tolerance. Blood and pancreata were extracted for analysis. Blood and pancreata were also collected from mice prior to the start of the diet regime, and prior to the start of drug treatment.

it is useful to have more than one method of assessment as well as quantitative ways for assessing pancreatitis. We chose to measure plasma amylase and lipase content, a method that is used in the clinic to detect pancreatitis. However, both enzymes can be cleared by the renal system and this may be problematic for early diagnosis of pan-creatitis. Immunohistochemistry gives the ability to detect early pan-creatic damage, provided the right markers are used. For example, we chose to assess Reg3b content as it is an indicator of tissue regenera-tion and is up-regulated when pancreata are damaged, e.g. by pan-creatitis. Thus, a change in the content of this protein in the pancreas can be a measure for mild pancreatitis, where pancreatic tissue is avail-able for analysis. The administered dose is obviously a consideration; this should be comparable to that used in humans. In model systems the administered dose is usually estimated by the weight of the ani-mal. Where high-fat diet is used, this raises the question of whether adipose versus muscle mass should be taken in to consideration for the calculation of drug dose. However, these measures of tissue mass are not currently straightforward to obtain for all researchers.

Sensitivity to drug doses is subject to strain and species differences, and this should be taken into consideration.

There are also differences in the route of administration of the treatment. For example, sitagliptin is normally administered orally. This is not particularly easy in rodent systems — oral gavage is a stressful procedure that is not practical on large cohorts on daily administration for long periods of time; administration by admixture is extremely costly and may limit the ability of researchers to conduct such research; and administration using gel pellets requires prior training of the animals and may incur problems such as taste aversion in prolonged treatment periods. It is possible to administer sitagliptin by intraperitoneal injection or through subcutaneously implanted minipumps; the required dose and efficacy of such methods need to be validated if they are not the normal route of administration in humans.

8.2.1.1. *Protocol summary*

1. Perform intraperitoneal glucose tolerance test (IPGTT) on eight-week-old mice and then place on high fat diet (60%) or normal chow. Monitor weight weekly till the end of the drug treatment period.
2. Perform IPGTT on mice eight weeks after start of diet regime to verify glucose intolerance has been effected in the high-fat-diet-fed cohort.
3. Start daily administration of saline, GLP-1R agonist or DPP-IV inhibitor by IP injection at the start of the dark phase. Assign mice such that each cage contains mice injected with each of the drugs, i.e. so that there are cage controls for each drug. Extract blood for plasma GLP-1 measurements to verify efficacy of drug treatment. Perform injections for 75 days.
4. Perform IPGTT on mice at the end of the drug treatment period to check for changes in glucose tolerance. Extract blood to measure amylase and lipase using commercially available kits.
5. Extract pancreata, fix in formalin, wax embed and cut into 5 μm sections. Stain slices with eosin and haematoxylin and send for histopathological analysis. Stain with antibodies to identify

specific cell populations (e.g. insulin and glucagon for islet cell types) and markers of pancreatitis (e.g. Reg3B), image using Widefield microscopy and quantify using Fiji (Image J; http://fiji.sc/Fiji). For histopathology and quantification of pancreatitis markers, blind the person performing the imaging and analysis by asking another researcher to re-label the slides with alternative nomenclature (e.g. by using a random number generator) to avoid bias.

8.3. Conclusions

Despite the recent publication of data indicating the requirement for caution in the use of GLP-1-based drugs, there are obvious advantages in this treatment modality, which makes the development and refinement of GLP-1-based treatment attractive. The incretin effect, mediated in part by GLP-1, is responsible for 20–80% of postprandial insulin secretion in a healthy individual. Another beneficial aspect of the GLP-1 pathway is its glucose dependency even in the constant presence of GLP-1R agonists, which allows for a decrease in the risk of hypoglycaemia in comparison to other treatment agents. The indirect mechanism involved in the inhibition of glucagon secretion is abolished at low glucose levels as well as the intracellular signalling leading to insulin exocytosis in the presence of GLP-1. Moreover, GLP-1 might be able to reverse glucose-resistance in β cells by increasing insulin biosynthesis to refill insulin stores, and restore glucose sensitivity in β cells through a surge in the expression of glucose transporters and glucokinase (see Chapter 3). Furthermore, a rise in GLP-1 signalling induces weight loss because of its effect on appetite and gastric emptying, which is useful in diabetic patients who are also obese; for these patients weight loss is accompanied by improved insulin sensitivity and slowing of the disease development. Moreover, GLP-1 is thought to preserve the function of β cells by exerting protective and proliferative effects, and this might therefore provide a method to slow down the progression of the disease.

However, as emphasised in this chapter, these proliferative effects of GLP-1 may also be a cause for concern. It is known that

GLP-1-based therapies induce acinar-to-ductal metaplasia and increase ductal, acinar and α cell proliferation, each of which can cause obstructions and inflammation due to misplacement of digestive enzymes (Fig. 8.4). Indeed, this may be the mechanism by which pancreatitis develops in patients taking these drugs. Another proposed mechanism by which GLP-1-based therapies may increase the risk of pancreatitis is through alterations in gastric emptying, which

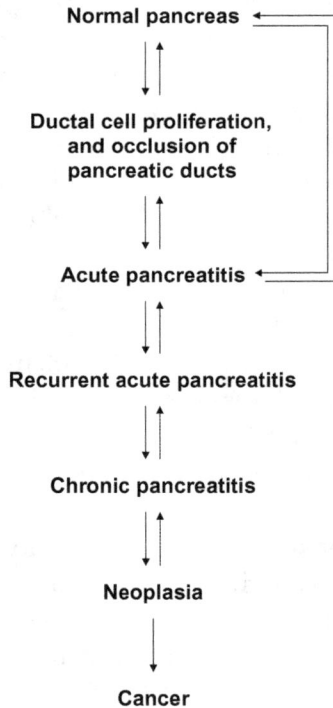

Figure 8.4. Potential mechanism whereby GLP-1 mimetics may lead to pancreatitis and pancreatic cancer. It has been proposed that administration of GLP-1 mimetics and DPP-IV inhibitors could lead to damage of the exocrine pancreas, potentially via pancreatic duct occlusion following ductal cell proliferation. This would result in acute pancreatitis that may be resolved by anti-inflammatory processes, but would result in fibrosis. Repeated insults would lead to recurrent acute pancreatitis, which may then become chronic and, in the long term, become neoplastic with additional DNA damage. Recovery from chronic pancreatitis and neoplasia may be incomplete, and may lead to cancer with further accumulation of damage.

lead to the increased chance of gallstones, the main risk factor for pancreatitis. As pancreatitis (even at sub-clinical levels) is a risk factor for pancreatic cancer, a major concern is the possible effect of GLP-1-based therapies on the risk for the latter disease. However, GLP-1-based therapies are often used in combination with other anti-diabetes therapeutics such as metformin (more commonly in Europe than in the US). Metformin is commonly used as a first-line treatment for T2D, but the progressive worsening of glycaemic control often seen in T2D patients requires additional treatment, e.g. combined treatment with metformin and sulfonylureas or GLP-1 receptor agonists. For example, only 45% of the patients in the intensive-control group in UKPDS (United Kingdom Prospective Diabetes Study) were able to maintain glycaemic control on metformin alone for three years. Importantly, metformin tends to exert anti-proliferative effects on cells, possibly through stimulating AMP (adenosine monophosphate)-activated protein kinase, and is known to lower cancer risk. The risk of hypoglycaemia and weight gain is low when metformin is used in combination with GLP-1R-agonist-based therapies, making metformin and GLP-1 mimetics a popular treatment combination. Future studies on long-term combined use of metformin and GLP-1 mimetics, in humans and in animal models with lesions that mimic the diabetic state in humans, may be useful to refine treatment modalities for patients with diabetes.

Another point worthy of note is the demonstration that liraglutide may increase the risk of thyroid cancer in rodent models. This was proposed to be due to increased calcitonin release from medullary C cells and was shown to be the case in rodent C cell lines but human C cell lines proved resistant to GLP-1-induced calcitonin release. The discrepancy in data from rodent and human C cell lines may be due to differences in GLP-1R expression between these cells. GLP-1R content in different thyroid cell types is currently under dispute. Whilst GLP-1R content in the human thyroid, and thus the potential for GLP-1 mimetics to induce thyroid cancer, is still unclear, it is perhaps prudent to be cautious in the administration of these drugs to people who may be at increased risk of developing medullary thyroid cancer. Also, a small proportion of patients develop antibodies against liraglutide and exenatide. The phenomena of immunotoxicity and anti-drug antibody response is one that has led to the failure of many peptide-based biopharmaceuticals to pass clinical trials. Immunogenicity may be induced by the intrinsic antigenicity of the T cell epitopes in the drug, or by extrinsic factors, e.g. the disease setting may predispose individuals to a higher or lower immune response. Antibodies are generated if the drug contains relevant helper T cell epitopes (11–20 amino acid sequence), which are then presented by human leukocyte antigen (HLA) class II molecules to CD4+ T cells, leading to the activation of the T cell's immune responses against the epitopes. For exenatide and liraglutide, the level of antibodies did not appear to be sufficient to interfere with glycaemic control, but it remains possible that therapeutic efficacy may be reduced in individuals with very high antibody levels. Antibodies against GLP-1 mimetics may also trigger adverse effects, ranging from mild injection site reactions to life-threatening anaphylaxis. Thus, constant surveillance for adverse effects in patients on these drugs is important, as is the development of GLP-1 mimetics that are more structurally similar to native GLP-1 (as these are less likely to induce antibody formation).

One cannot leave this discussion without mentioning the public's interest in the dispute. A likely outcome is that patients may be more wary of these drugs, and may want more discussion with their physicians if these were prescribed. This in itself may not be detrimental, as patient interest and vigilance in their own treatment are positive outcomes. However, there may be adverse effects on adherence to therapy, which may negatively impact patient health. On a wider scale, the public are now more aware of the drug testing process and the (lack of) availability/publication of results from drug tests. There was also criticism over the slow response of the European and American drug regulators to the concerns raised about these drugs. This is in line with the public's growth of interest in their medical treatment, with the general increase in the availability of information on the internet. In general, we consider openness and greater transparency to be good things. Health care professionals and scientists need to be more prepared to engage in such discussions with the general public.

References

1. Drucker, D.J., Sherman, S.I., Bergenstal, R.M. and Buse, J.B. (2011). The safety of incretin-based therapies — review of the scientific evidence, *J. Clin. Endocrinol. Metab.*, **96**, 2027–2031.
2. Labuzek, K., Kozlowski, M., Szkudlapski, D., Sikorska, P., Kozlowska, M. and Okopien, B. (2013). Incretin-based therapies in the treatment of type 2 diabetes — more than meets the eye?, *Eur. J. Intern. Med.*, **24**, 207–212.
3. Nauck, M.A. and Friedrich, N. (2013). Do GLP-1-based therapies increase cancer risk?, *Diabetes Care*, **36**(Suppl 2), S245–S252.
4. Lowenfels, A.B., Maisonneuve, P., Cavallini, G., Ammann, R.W., Lankisch, P.G., Andersen, J.R., Dimagno, E.P., Andrén-Sandberg, A. and Domellöf, L. (1993). Pancreatitis and the risk of pancreatic cancer, International Pancreatitis Study Group, *N. Engl. J. Med.*, **328**, 1433–1437.
5. Jura, N., Archer, H. and Bar-Sagi, D. (2005). Chronic pancreatitis, pancreatic adenocarcinoma and the black box in-between, *Cell Res.*, **15**, 72–77.
6. Bhanot, U.K. and Moller, P. (2009). Mechanisms of parenchymal injury and signaling pathways in ectatic ducts of chronic pancreatitis: Implications for pancreatic carcinogenesis, *Lab. Invest.*, **89**, 489–497.
7. Elashoff, M., Matveyenko, A.V., Gier, B., Elashoff, R. and Butler, P.C. (2011). Pancreatitis, pancreatic, and thyroid cancer with glucagon-like peptide-1-based therapies, *Gastroenterology*, **141**, 150–156.
8. Ellenbroek, J.H., Tons, H.A., Westerouen van Meeteren, M.J., de Graaf, N., Hanegraaf, M.A., Rabelink, T.J., Carlotti, F. and de Koning, E.J. (2013). Glucagon-like peptide-1 receptor agonist treatment reduces beta cell mass in normoglycaemic mice, *Diabetologia*, **56**, 1980–1986.
9. van der Worp, H.B., Howells, D.W., Sena, E.S., Porritt, M.J., Rewell, S., O'Collins, V. and Macleod, M.R. (2010). Can animal models of disease reliably inform human studies?, *PLoS Med.*, **7**, e1000245.
10. Mondragon, A., Davidsson, D., Kyriakidou, S., Bertling, A., Gomes-Faria, R., Cohen, P., Rothery, S., Chabosseau, P., Rutter, G.A. and da Silva Xavier, G. (2014). Divergent effects of liraglutide, exendin-4, and sitagliptin on beta-cell mass and indicators of pancreatitis in a mouse model of hyperglycaemia, *PLoS One*, **9**(8), e104873.

Index